Managing Symptoms in the Pharmacy

FASTtrack

Managing
Symptoms
in the Pharmacy

Alan Nathan
Freelance pharmacy writer and consultant
London, UK

Pharmaceutical Press
London • Chicago

Published by the Pharmaceutical Press
An imprint of RPS Publishing
1 Lambeth High Street, London SE1 7JN, UK
100 South Atkinson Road, Suite 200, Grayslake, IL 60030-7820, USA

© Pharmaceutical Press 2008

(**PP**)is a trade mark of RPS Publishing
RPS Publishing is the publishing organisation of the Royal Pharmaceutical
Society of Great Britain

First published 2008

Design and layout by Designers Collective, London
Printed in Great Britain by TJ International, Padstow, Cornwall

ISBN 978 0 85369 727 5

A catalogue record for this book is available from the British Library.

Contents

Introduction to the *FASTtrack* series   vii
About the author   viii

1. Introduction **1**
    Features of this book   1

Cardiovascular
2. Cardiovascular conditions **7**
    Myocardial infarction
    (MI, heart attack)   7
    Angina pectoris   8
    Heart failure (HF)   9
    Stroke   10

Central nervous system
3. Motion sickness **17**
4. Pain **21**
    Headache and migraine   21
    Dental pain   28

Eye and ear
5. Ear problems **33**
    Earache   33
    Ear wax   33
    Otitis externa   34
6. Eye conditions **37**
    Conditions of the cornea   37
    Conditions of the eyelid   40
    Other eye problems   42

Foot conditions
7. Athlete's foot **47**
8. Foot (podiatric) problems **53**
    Hard and soft corns and calluses   53
    Bunions   55
    Ingrown toenail   56
9. Fungal nail infection
(onychomycosis). **57**
10. Verrucas (plantar warts) and warts
(common warts). **61**

Gastrointestinal
11. Constipation **67**
12. Diarrhoea **75**
13. Haemorrhoids (piles). **83**
14. Irritable-bowel syndrome (IBS) **89**

15. Indigestion **93**
16. Mouth ulcers
(minor aphthous ulcers). **101**

Infestations
17. Head lice **107**
18. Scabies **113**
19. Threadworm **117**

Musculoskeletal
20. Musculoskeletal conditions **123**
    Sports injuries   123
    Back pain   125
21. Common cold and influenza. **131**
    Sore throat   134
22. Cough. **139**
23. Hayfever. **147**
24. Nicotine replacement therapy
(NRT) **155**

Skin
25. Acne. **163**
26. Cold sores (oral herpes simplex) . . . **169**
27 Eczema/dermatitis **173**
28. Fungal skin infections **179**
    Tinea corporosis (ringworm)   180
    Tinea cruris (dhobie itch, jock itch)   180
    Pityriasis versicolor   181
29. Scalp conditions **183**
    Dandruff   183
    Seborrhoeic dermatitis   185
    Cradle cap   186
    Scalp psoriasis   187
    Scalp ringworm (tinea capitis)   187

Women's conditions
30. Cystitis. **193**
31. Dysmenorrhoea. **197**
32. Emergency hormonal contraception
(EHC) **203**
33. Premenstrual syndrome (PMS) **207**
34. Vaginal thrush. **211**

Answers to self-assessment   215
Glossary   227
Index   229

Introduction to the
FASTtrack series

FASTtrack is a new series of revision guides created for undergraduate pharmacy students. The books are intended to be used in conjunction with textbooks and reference books as an aid to revision to help guide students through their exams. They provide essential information required in each particular subject area. The books will also be useful for pre-registration trainees preparing for the Royal Pharmaceutical Society of Great Britain's (RPSGB's) registration examination, and to practising pharmacists as a quick reference text.

The content of each title focuses on what pharmacy students really need to know in order to pass exams. Features include*:
- concise bulleted information
- key points
- tips for the student
- multiple-choice questions (MCQs) and worked examples
- case studies
- simple diagrams.

The titles in the *FASTtrack* series reflect the full spectrum of modules for the undergraduate pharmacy degree.

Titles include:
Pharmaceutical Compounding and Dispensing
Physical Pharmacy (based on Florence & Attwood's *Physicochemical Principles of Pharmacy*)
Pharmaceutics: Dosage Form and Design
Pharmaceutics: Delivery and Targeting
Therapeutics
Complementary and Alternative Therapies

There is also an accompanying website which includes extra MCQs, further title information and sample content: www.fasttrackpharmacy.com.

If you have any feedback regarding this series, please contact us at feedback@fasttrackpharmacy.com.

*Note: not all features are in every title in the series.

About the author

After qualifying, ALAN NATHAN was a lecturer in pharmacognosy at Sunderland School of Pharmacy for 2 years, before spending the next 23 years as a community pharmacist, 14 of these as an independent proprietor. In 1989, he was appointed Boots Teacher/Practitioner in the Department of Pharmacy, King's College, London and became a full-time lecturer in pharmacy practice there in 1994. In 2004, he retired from King's College to become a freelance pharmacy writer and consultant.

Alan has published widely in pharmacy and other health profession journals, his main areas of interest being the treatment of minor ailments, and pharmacy law and ethics.

Alan was also a member of the Council of the Royal Pharmaceutical Society from 1986 until 2002, and is co-founder and chairman of the Society's Listening Friends stress help scheme for pharmacists.

chapter 1
Introduction

Features of this book

This book contains all the essential information required for managing symptoms presented in the pharmacy, and covers the common ailments that pharmacists are likely to be presented with. Each chapter is set out in the same structured format and content is presented concisely in a bullet-point form, for quick reference and to make the information easy to understand, assimilate and memorise.

The main features of the book are as follows:

Symptom management

- The book deals with the minor illnesses or conditions that can be self-treated with advice and treatment from a pharmacist. Three chapters deal with medicines (Chapter 24, nicotine replacement therapy; Chapter 32, emergency hormonal contraception; and Chapter 2, simvastatin) that have become available without prescription within the last few years and are not treatments for illnesses but are used prophylactically or preventively.
- The book is organised into 34 chapters, arranged in 10 sections based on body systems (e.g. respiratory) or types of condition (e.g. fungal infections), plus a section dealing with women's conditions that includes a chapter on emergency hormonal contraception (Chapter 32).
- Each chapter on illnesses is structured in the same way, to provide a systematic approach and facilitate learning, under the following headings (the three chapters on medicines have a slightly different but equally structured format):
- Causes – to provide an understanding of how a condition comes about
- Epidemiology – to give an indication of the incidence and prevalence of a condition, as an aid to diagnosis
- Symptoms and signs – the common presenting symptoms, and signs that can be observed by a pharmacist, that characterise a condition
- Differential diagnosis – conditions with similar features to the minor illness being considered, but that are more serious and would require referral for further investigation
- Symptoms, signs and circumstances for referral – features indicating the need for referral to another health professional
- Treatment:
  - a summary of prescription treatments for a condition, where available
  - details of the non-prescription treatments for a condition
- Further advice – advice a pharmacist can give to help minimise the effects, or prevent recurrence, of a condition

- Case study – a presentation of a scenario, providing readers with an opportunity to apply the information in the chapter and use problem-solving skills to deal with typical situations and queries presented in the community pharmacy.

Exam help and advice

Each chapter contains:

- tips for students and pre-registration trainees on exam technique and how to maximise their chances of passing
- multiple choice questions based on the information in the chapter, in the formats used in the Royal Pharmaceutical Society of Great Britain registration exam.

A brief explanation of the registration exam and questions

Structure of the registration examination

- There are two papers:
- 'closed-book': 90 questions to be answered from memory (no references allowed) in 1½ hours
- 'open-book': 80 questions to be answered in 2½ hours, using the *British National Formulary*, *Medicines Ethics and Practice* and the *Drug Tariff* as references. The paper includes a 20-question calculations section, which must be answered without a calculator.
- The pass mark is a 70% average over the two papers (including 70% in the calculations section of the open-book paper), but with no minimum pass mark for the individual papers.

Question formats

Four types of question are used:

1. Simple completion: the question is followed by five suggested answers, and the best answer must be selected. The following is an example:

Mrs L's dose of methotrexate is adjusted according to response. Which one of the following is the maximum dose of methotrexate that Mrs L could be given?

a. 7.5 mg weekly
b. 10 mg weekly
c 12.5 mg weekly
d. 20 mg weekly
e. 25 mg weekly

2. Multiple completion: three options are presented, one or more of which is correct. After deciding which is or are correct, one of the following is chosen:

a. if all three are correct
b. if the first two only are correct
c. if the last two only are correct
d. if only the first is correct
e. if only the last is correct

Example
The following patients are admitted to hospital suffering from invasive salmonellosis. Your hospital's antibiotic policy states that ciprofloxacin is the antibiotic of choice for this condition unless cautioned due to a pre-existing medical condition or interaction. It would be appropriate for you to advise that ciprofloxacin should be used with caution in which of these patients?
1.   a woman who has asthma
2.   a man who takes digoxin
3.   a woman who has epilepsy

3.   Classification: groups of 2–4 questions, consisting of three to five lettered headings, are followed by a list of numbered questions. For each numbered question the one heading which is most closely related to it is selected. Each heading may be used once, more than once, or not at all.
Example
Questions 1–4 concern the following antibiotics:
a.   oxytetracycline
b.   flucloxacillin
c.   metronidazole
d.   ciprofloxacin
e.   sodium fusidate
Select from (a) to (e) which one of the above antibiotics:
1.   would be an appropriate treatment for a patient with pseudomembranous colitis
2.   is usually given with a second antibiotic to prevent the emergence of resistance
3.   is active against Pseudomonas
4.   can be given by the rectal route as an effective alternative to intravenous therapy when oral administration is not possible

4.   Assertion/reason: questions consist of two statements. After deciding whether the first statement is true or false and whether the second statement is true or false, the following options are chosen:
a.   if both statements are true and the second statement is a correct explanation of the first statement
b.   if both statements are true but the second statement is not a correct explanation of the first statement
c.   if the first statement is true but the second statement is false
d.   if the first statement is false but the second statement is true
e.   if both statements are false
Example
Question 1 concerns the following scenario:
Mrs E has endocarditis and has been prescribed gentamicin 80 mg tds. A pre-dose serum level is taken and found to be 1.5 mg/l.

First statement: Mrs E's dose of gentamicin should be reduced.
Second statement: The pre-dose serum concentration for gentamicin for the treatment of endocarditis should be less than 1 mg/l.

Answers

The last section in the book gives suggested answers to the case studies and answers to the multiple choice questions, with rationales for answers where necessary.

References

British National Formulary, no. 54. London: BMJ Publishing Group/RPS Publishing, 2007.
Drug Tariff. London: The Stationery Office. Also available online at: www.ppa.org.uk.
Medicines Ethics and Practice, no. 31. London: Royal Pharmaceutical Society of Great Britain, 2007.

Cardiovascular

chapter 2
Cardiovascular conditions

In general the diagnosis and treatment of cardiovascular diseases are the domain of medical practitioners. However, there is some scope for the involvement of pharmacists in this area beyond the dispensing of prescribed medication, because:

- some medicines for the prevention of cardiovascular disease are available without prescription
- pharmacists may be able to recognise some of the early signs of cardiovascular disease and refer patients for investigation and treatment before a condition becomes critical
- pharmacists may be required to provide assistance to patients with cardiovascular conditions who are taken ill in the pharmacy or are brought in for emergency aid.

This chapter provides relevant clinical features of the main cardiovascular conditions and information about medicines available without prescription for their prevention.

Myocardial infarction (MI, heart attack)
Causes

- MI is essentially the death of myocardial tissue, caused by an insufficiency of oxygen supply to the myocardium.
- It usually results from rupture of an atheromatous plaque in a coronary vessel, leading to thrombus formation, blocking the vessel and causing occlusion of the vessel and myocardial ischaemia.
- Heart muscle begins to die within 20–40 minutes if blood flow is not restored, and necrosis is irreversible if the coronary vessel remains occluded for more than 4–6 hours.

Epidemiology

- Average UK incidence of MI is about 1 in 200 in the population per year.
- Relative incidence in men and women is about 2.2:1.
- Mortality is about 25%, and half of those who die never reach hospital.

Symptoms and warning signs

- Central chest pain or sensations of severe pressure, fullness, squeezing or discomfort:

- – lasting for more than a few minutes
- – of increasing intensity
- – radiating to the shoulders, neck, arms or jaw
- – not relieved by rest or cardiac medication
- ▪ with any or all of the following:
- – sweating or cool, clammy skin
- – skin pallor and/or bluish lips
- – shortness of breath
- – nausea or vomiting
- – dizziness or fainting
- – rapid or irregular pulse
- – anxiety.

Differential diagnosis

Chest pain may be a symptom of indigestion, pleurisy, pneumonia or other disorders, but the duration, severity of pain, intensity of distress and accompanying symptoms of an MI leave little doubt that, whatever the cause, the situation is an emergency.

Emergency aid

- ▪ Put patient into a half-sitting position, with head and shoulders supported (e.g. with cushions or pillows) and knees bent.
- ▪ Dial 999 for an ambulance.
- ▪ Help patients to use any angina medication they are carrying.
- ▪ If patient is fully conscious, give a 300 mg aspirin tablet to chew.
- ▪ Monitor breathing and pulse rate and be prepared to give mouth-to-mouth ventilation and chest compressions if necessary.

Angina pectoris
Causes

- ▪ Angina occurs when myocardial demand for oxygen exceeds the ability of the coronary arteries to supply oxygenated blood. The cause is usually coronary artery obstruction due to atherosclerosis.
- ▪ The most common form of the condition is stable angina. It is brought on by physical exertion or other forms of stress, including exposure to cold, heavy meals or intense emotion, and is relieved by rest.
- ▪ Unstable angina is a syndrome of attacks of increasing frequency and severity, occurring on minimal exertion or at rest. It often leads to MI.

Epidemiology

About 1.2 million people in the UK have or have had angina – 9% of men and 5% of women aged 55–64, and 14% of men and 8% of women aged 65–74.

Symptoms and warning signs

- The patient may experience a sensation in the centre of the chest variously described as pressure, fullness, squeezing, tightness, burning or a heavy weight.
- It may also manifest as pain in the epigastric region, back or jaw, and may radiate to the shoulders, neck or arms.
- Pain ranges in intensity from mild to severe.
- Other symptoms, as occur with MI (see above), may be experienced.
- Unlike MI, pain is reversible on rest; attacks last only a few minutes and are relieved by coronary vasodilators.

Differential diagnosis

As for MI, but may be more difficult to distinguish from other conditions causing pain and other symptoms in the chest and epigastric region.

Emergency aid

- Sit the person down in a quiet area, make the patient comfortable and reassure.
- Allow the person to use any coronary vasodilator medication he or she is carrying. (If the individual has no medication but confirms that he or she has angina, you may give a glyceryl trinitrate tablet or similar medication.)
- Allow the person to rest until the attack is over.

Heart failure (HF)
Causes

- HF describes a usually gradual weakening in heart tissue and a decline in its ability to perform its function to pump blood around the body.
- There are several causes:
- reduced ventricular contractility, as result of myocarditis (inflammation of the myocardium), cardiomyopathy (hypertrophy of heart tissue) or MI
- ventricular outflow obstruction, caused by hypertension, narrowing of the aorta (aortic stenosis), pulmonary hypertension or pulmonary valve stenosis
- ventricular inflow obstruction, as a result of stenosis of the mitral and tricuspid valves, among other causes
- ventricular volume overload, due to failure of the mitral valve regulating the flow of blood into the left ventricle and the septa separating the heart chambers
- arrhythmias.

Epidemiology

- HF is a disease of the elderly – average age at first diagnosis is 76 years.
- Incidence is increasing with increasing life expectancy and higher survival rates following MI.
- About 1 in 35 people aged 65–74 years have HF, increasing to about 1 in 15 of those aged 75–84 years, and to 1 in 7 in those over 85.

Symptoms and warning signs

- fatigue and shortness of breath after mild exertion
- a dry, wheezy, hacking cough occurring a few hours after lying down but stopping after sitting up
- when there is pulmonary oedema, there may be a cough producing a pinkish froth
- accumulation of fluid in the feet, ankles, legs and abdomen
- weight loss.

Emergency aid

- Pharmacists would not normally encounter situations of acute HF, which often occur at night. Symptoms include severe breathlessness, often accompanied by MI symptoms.
- Emergency aid is as for MI.

Stroke
Causes

- Stroke is caused by the death of brain cells as a result of interruption of blood flow to them, causing permanent disability.
- 80% occur as a consequence of ischaemia, caused either by a thrombus formed inside a cerebral artery as a result of arteriosclerosis, or an embolism formed elsewhere in the body and carried to the brain.
- 20% of strokes are accounted for by intracerebral haemorrhage due to rupture of a blood vessel, producing a clot displacing normal brain tissue and disrupting function.
- Transient ischaemic attacks (TIAs, 'ministrokes') last between a few minutes and a few hours, followed by complete recovery.

Epidemiology

- Stroke is the third most common cause of death in the UK and accounts for 12% of all deaths.
- Incidence increases markedly with age, and each year about 3% of the population over the age of 70 suffer a stroke.
- Stroke affects women more than men in a ratio of 2:1.

Symptoms and warning signs

- difficulty speaking or understanding speech (aphasia)
- difficulty walking
- vertigo
- numbness, paralysis or weakness, usually on one side of the body
- seizure (relatively rare)
- severe headache
- sudden confusion

- sudden decrease in the level of consciousness
- sudden loss of balance or coordination
- sudden vision problems (e.g. blurred vision, blindness in one eye)
- vomiting.

Emergency aid

- For someone who is conscious:
- lay the individual down with head and shoulders slightly raised and supported. Incline the patient's head to one side and place a towel or cloth on the shoulder to absorb any dribbling
- dial 999 for an ambulance.
- If unconscious:
- maintain an open airway, and be prepared to resuscitate if necessary
- loosen any clothing that might impede breathing
- call an ambulance.

Non-prescription medicines for the prevention of cardiovascular disease

Simvastatin

- Simvastatin is one of a group of drugs known as statins that act by competitively inhibiting 3-hydroxy-3-methylglutaryl coenzyme A (HMG-CoA) reductase, the enzyme that mediates cholesterol synthesis in the liver.
- Inhibition of HMG-CoA increases the formation of low-density lipoprotein (LDL) receptors on hepatocyte membranes, leading to increased clearance of LDL cholesterol and reduction in total serum cholesterol.
- The main biochemical effect of the statins is to lower LDL cholesterol, but they also raise levels of high-density lipoprotein (HDL) cholesterol, which improves the HDL:LDL cholesterol ratio (a more important index than total serum cholesterol), and they also reduce plasma triglycerides.
- Statins have been shown to be safe and effective in lowering cholesterol, and it has been recommended that a statin should be prescribed as secondary prevention for all patients with symptomatic cardiovascular disease.
- Statins have also been recommended for all people without symptoms but who are considered to be at moderate risk (i.e. 10–15% risk of developing coronary heart disease (CHD) within the next 10 years); it is possible to determine moderate risk through self-reported risk factors.

Licensed indications

- For sale as a P medicine, simvastatin 10 mg at a dose of one 10 mg tablet each night, on a long-term basis is indicated to reduce the risk of a first major coronary event in individuals at moderate risk of CHD, including:
- men aged 55–70, with or without risk factors
- men aged 45–54, with one or more listed risk factors
- postmenopausal women aged 55–70, with one or more risk factors.

- ▪ The risk factors are:
- – smoker – currently or within the last 5 years
- – family history of CHD – father or a brother had a heart attack before age 55, or mother or a sister before age 65
- – overweight or obese – body mass index above 25, or waist measurement greater than 100 cm (40 in) in men or 87.5 cm (35 in) in women
- – South-Asian family origin.

Licensing restrictions

Over-the-counter simvastatin is considered not suitable in the following circumstances for the following people, who should be referred to a doctor:

- ▪ men over 55 years with a family history of CHD and at least one other risk factor, as above
- ▪ people with, or reporting, any symptoms that might suggest: any cardiovascular, cerebrovascular or peripheral vascular disorder; liver disease or history of abnormal liver function tests; renal impairment; hypothyroidism; myopathy or family history of muscle disorders
- ▪ people with a known fasting LDL-cholesterol level of 5.5 mmol/l or above (cholesterol testing before sale is not a licensing requirement but is recommended as good practice by the Royal Pharmaceutical Society of Great Britain (RPSGB))
- ▪ people whose blood pressure is known and within the range for referral in accordance with RPSGB practice guidance (blood pressure testing before sale is not a licensing requirement but is recommended as good practice by the RPSGB)
- ▪ men who consume more than 4 units and women who consume more than 3 units of alcohol per day, and people who drink more than 1 litre grapefruit juice per day
- ▪ people who have suffered previous side-effects or allergy when taking cholesterol-lowering medication.

RPSGB good practice recommendations

In addition to the licensing conditions, the RPSGB recommends the following good-practice measures in association with the over-the-counter sale of simvastatin:

- ▪ Pharmacists should be involved in all initial sales but subsequent sales may be delegated to appropriately trained medicines counter assistants.
- ▪ Where possible, sales should be recorded in the patient's medication record.
- ▪ Lifestyle advice to reduce the risk of CHD should be given to purchasers.
- ▪ Pharmacists should liaise with local general practitioners and primary-care organisations to fit in with local policies on management of CHD risk and prescribing of statins; they should encourage purchasers to inform their general practitioner that they are taking simvastatin.
- ▪ Pharmacists should monitor people who buy simvastatin at least once a year for adverse effects, interactions, changes in risk factors and blood cholesterol levels.

Adverse effects

- Simvastatin is generally well tolerated and side-effects are usually rare, mild and transient.
- Myopathy and rhabdomyolisis, characterised by generalised muscle pain, tenderness or weakness, have been reported very rarely.
- Liver dysfunction, gastrointestinal disturbances and hypersensitivity reactions have also been reported rarely.

Interactions

- Simvastatin is metabolised in the liver by the P450 isoenzyme CYP3A4 and interactions can occur with drugs that inhibit this enzyme.
- Simvastatin may also increase the anticoagulant effect of warfarin and other coumarins.
- Drugs that can cause myopathy or rhabdomyolysis, including fibric acid derivatives and nicotinic acid, increase the risk of developing these conditions if given in association with simvastatin.

Low-dose aspirin

- Low-dose aspirin reduces the risk of MI, increases survival in patients who have had an acute MI and reduces the risk of stroke, through inhibiting thrombus formation within coronary and cerebral blood vessels.
- The anti-inflammatory and antithrombotic effects of aspirin depend on its ability to inactivate the enzyme cyclo-oxygenase. Platelets (thrombocytes) in the blood play an important role in the process of coagulation. Through irreversible inhibition of cyclo-oxygenase, aspirin prevents the synthesis of thromboxane A_2 which promotes platelet adhesion and aggregation. Platelets cannot synthesise more thromboxane A_2, which is only restored when existing platelets are replaced from the vascular endothelium. Continuous low dosing with aspirin thereby maintains thromboxane A_2 at a low level.
- Antiplatelet aspirin is indicated for the secondary prevention of thrombotic cerebrovascular and cardiovascular disease, at a dose of 75 mg daily.
- Low-dose aspirin is also indicated for primary prevention of MI or stroke when the estimated 10-year cardiovascular disease risk is 20% or greater.
- Antiplatelet aspirin therapy should only be initiated on the advice of a doctor.
- The same contraindications, cautions and interactions apply as for aspirin at analgesic doses.

Omega-3 triglycerides

- Omega-3 triglycerides are derived from fish oils. They contain triglycerides of omega-3 fatty acids, particularly eicosapentaenoic acid (EPA) and docosahexaenoic acid (DHA). These exert an antithrombotic effect by competing with arachidonic acid for inclusion in cyclo-oxygenase and lipoxygenase synthesis pathways, reducing platelet aggregation and decreasing platelet counts. They also lower blood cholesterol levels through reduction of very-low-density-lipoproteins. As cyclo-oxygenase inhibitors they also have anti-inflammatory activity.

- EPA and DHA in fish oil have a role in the secondary prevention of cardiovascular disease.
- Almost all products containing fish oils are marketed as food supplements, not medicines.

Self-assessment

Case study

A man wants to buy simvastatin tablets because he says he wants to keep his cholesterol down. On questioning he tells you he is 40 years old. His body mass index, which you calculate from the weight and height measurements he gives you, is 22. He says that he is worried about having a heart attack, because he has a high-powered and stressful job and his father, who was born in India, had a heart attack at the age of 56. He says he had an annual health check recently and that no problems were identified and his cholesterol level was 5.2 mmol/l. He is a non-smoker.

Would you sell him the simvastatin tablets, or what action would you take?.

Multiple choice questions

1. (Open-book, multiple completion)
   A general practitioner wants to prescribe simvastatin to a patient who is already taking several drugs and wants to know if there is likely to be a clinically significant interaction with any of them. With which of the following is there the possibility of a potentially hazardous interaction?
   a. Aspirin 75 mg
   b. Amiodarone
   c. Verapamil

2. (Open-book, multiple completion)
   Which of the following packs of generic aspirin tablets 75 mg can be sold in any retail outlet?
   a. 28 dispersible tablets
   b. 28 enteric-coated tablets
   c. 28 standard tablets

3. (Open-book, multiple completion)
   Which of the following could only be supplied against a prescription?
   a. 1 × 56 aspirin dispersible tablets 75 mg
   b. 1 × 56 aspirin enteric-coated tablets 75 mg
   c. 1 × 56 aspirin standard tablets 75 mg

Tips

In the registration examination make sure you answer all questions on both papers – you cannot get marks for questions you do not answer, and there is no negative marking, so you will not be penalised for an incorrect answer.

Central
nervous system

Motion sickness	17
Pain	21

chapter 3
Motion sickness

Causes

- Motion sickness is a form of vertigo in which autonomic symptoms predominate.
- The cause is thought to be disturbance of the vestibular apparatus of the inner ear, which controls balance, brought on by unaccustomed types of movement. During travel conflicting stimuli are received in the brain from the eyes and remembered experience of usual forms of movement, such as walking. This sensory mismatch is interpreted as a noxious stimulus and initiates a physiological response similar to that to substances perceived as poisonous, and a number of autonomic nervous system responses are activated to reject the perceived poison.
- The body adapts to unfamiliar types of motion on prolonged or repeated exposure, explaining why seasickness, for example, tends to subside after a few days.

Epidemiology

- Motion sickness is more common in women than men.
- It is uncommon in children under 2 years and most common in children between 2 and 12, reaching a peak at 12 years. Incidence reduces thereafter and after 21 declines significantly with age.
- Women are more susceptible during menstruation and pregnancy.

Signs and symptoms

- Muscarinic effects, including:
- nausea
- vomiting
- increased salivation
- general malaise
- pallor
- sweating
- yawning
- hyperventilation.
- Gastric motility is also reduced and digestion impaired.

Differential diagnosis

- Nausea and vomiting occur in a wide range of conditions, but the symptoms of motion sickness are usually very clearly associated with travel. Patients will nearly always ask for advice on prevention rather than treatment of current symptoms.

Treatment

- Sedating antihistamines and hyoscine are licensed for use without prescription for prophylaxis and treatment of motion sickness. They appear to be of more or less equivalent efficacy.
- They are effective for prevention, but use for treatment is often unsuccessful as vomiting and gastric stasis prevent or substantially reduce their absorption.

Hyoscine

- Hyoscine competitively inhibits the actions of acetylcholine at the muscarinic receptors of autonomic effector sites innervated by parasympathetic nerves. It has a central as well as a peripheral action, as it is lipid-soluble and crosses the blood–brain barrier.
- Hyoscine is relatively short-acting and has more pronounced antimuscarinic side-effects than antihistamines (Table 3.1).

Table 3.1 Comparison of medications used in the treatment of seasickness

Drug	Efficacy	Drowsiness	Antimuscarinic side-effects	Length of action (hours)
Hyoscine	+++	+	+++	4
Antihistamines				
Cinnarizine	++	++	+	8
Meclozine	++	+	+	24
Promethazine hydrochloride	++	+++	++	6–8
Promethazine teoclate	++	++	++	24

Sedating antihistamines

- The older (first-generation) antihistamines which tend to cause sedation have antimuscarinic side-effects similar to the actions of hyoscine. (Second-generation antihistamines, which generally do not cause drowsiness, do not exert antimuscarinic side-effects and are of no use for motion sickness.)
- Sedating antihistamines licensed for the treatment of motion sickness (all P medicines) are:
- cinnarizine
- meclozine
- promethazine hydrochloride
- promethazine teoclate.
- The length of action, degree of sedation and side-effects vary between the antihistamines (Table 3.1)

Side-effects and cautions: hyoscine and antihistamines

- Hyoscine and antihistamines exhibit the same range of side-effects. However, side-effects tend to be more pronounced with hyoscine, and include:
- dry mouth
- blurred vision
- urinary retention
- constipation
- sedation (more marked with antihistamines).
- Both hyoscine and antihistamines should be avoided in patients suffering from glaucoma or prostatic hypertrophy, are not recommended for use by pregnant or breastfeeding women, and should be used with caution in the elderly and patients with epilepsy or cardiac or cardiovascular disease.
- Hyoscine and sedating antihistamines increase the effects of other drugs that cause sedation or have antimuscarinic actions, including many antidepressants and antipsychotic agents.
- Alcohol should be avoided when taking medication against motion sickness.

Additional advice

There are several things that people can do to minimise the chance of suffering from motion sickness on journeys.

General
- Avoid heavy meals before travelling.
- Avoid pungent odours.
- Avoid alcohol.

Road travel
- Drive, if possible, as drivers very rarely suffer from motion sickness.
- If you do not or cannot drive, sit in the front passenger seat if possible.
- Sit near the front in a bus or coach.
- Keep vehicle windows open.
- Do not try to read, and keep looking out of the window. Distract children with games such as I Spy, to make them look out.
- Listen to the radio or talk with other passengers.

Sea travel
- If possible, stay on deck and keep eyes fixed on the horizon.
- Below deck, stay in the centre of the ship and lie down with eyes closed.

Air travel
- Try to sit by the wing.

Self-assessment

Case study

A regular patient of yours tells you she is going on holiday to New Zealand and wants something to make sure that she does not get travel sickness on the long flight, but wants to be sure that whatever you recommend won't react badly with her prescribed medicines (perindopril and bendroflumethiazide for hypertension). She says that she doesn't want anything that will make her feel groggy, or that she has to take too often during the journey. She says that she usually takes cinnarizine, but wonders if there is anything better. She read in a magazine about ginger being good for travel sickness and wants to know what you think about it.

Multiple choice questions

1. (Open-book, multiple completion)
   Which of the following may be sold for the prevention of motion sickness?
   a. Valoid tablets for an 8-year-old child
   b. Phenergan elixir for a 2-year-old child
   c. Stugeron tablets for a 6-year-old child

2. (Open-book, simple completion)
   Which one of the following should not be sold for the prevention of motion sickness?
   a. Avomine tablets for a 5-year-old child
   b. Phenergan elixir for a 1-year-old child
   c. Phenergan 10 mg tablets for a 6-year-old child
   d. Stugeron tablets for a 6-year-old child
   e. Valoid tablets for an 8-year-old child

Tips

If you feel that you may have underperformed in the registration examination because of an unforeseen, serious adverse event, inform the RPSGB immediately. If you wait until after the result and find you have failed, an appeal is almost certain to be unsuccessful.

chapter 4
Pain

Headache and migraine
Causes

The causes of most headaches fall into three categories:

1. Tension: the most common cause of headache, thought to be due to pericranial muscle contraction. It is often psychogenic in origin and caused or made worse by tension, anxiety or fatigue.
2. Vascular, caused by dilatation or constriction of blood vessels in the brain and cranium: headaches associated with febrile illnesses are caused by vasodilatation. Migraine is also believed to be vascular in origin, at least in part, although neurochemical pathology also appears to be involved.
3. Traction: inflammation or compression of the brain and associated structures is responsible for headache associated with meningitis, encephalitis, haematomas (including those resulting from head injury), tumours and cerebral abscesses. Sinusitis, often associated with upper respiratory tract infections and allergic rhinitis, also frequently causes headache from congestion in the frontal and maxillary sinuses exerting pressure on surrounding nerves.

Other causes include:

- spasm or fatigue of the ciliary and periorbital muscles of the eye, causing eye strain
- glaucoma
- referred pain from the jaw; muscle strain and pulled ligaments in the neck or upper back
- inflammation of the temporal arteries in temporal arteritis
- neuropathic pain from shingles.

Epidemiology

- Headache is the most commonly experienced of all symptoms: 96% of people are estimated to suffer a headache at least once in their life and 80–90% will experience one or more per year.
- Migraine is suffered by about 15% of the population overall, with a female: male ratio of incidence of 3:1. Migraine mainly affects younger people: 80% of sufferers have their first attack before the age of 30, and incidence is rare after age 50.

Signs and symptoms

The clinical features of the main types of headache are outlined in Table 4.1.

Table 4.1 Clinical features of headache

Feature or symptom		Possible indication
Frequency/timing	Recurrent: associated with menstrual cycle or at certain times, e.g. weekends	Migraine
Location	Unilateral	Migraine (70% of cases)
	Bilateral (frontal/occipital)	Tension headache
	Bilateral (frontal)	Sinusitis
Type/severity	Mild/moderate, dull, 'like a band round the head'	Tension headache
	Moderate/severe, throbbing	Migraine
	Severe/intense ache or throbbing	Haemorrhage or aneurysm?
Duration	Few hours to 3 days	Migraine
	Few hours to (rarely) several days	Tension headache
Triggers/associated factors	Certain foods	Migraine
	Prodrome and visual/ neurological aura	Classical migraine (experienced by 25% of migraine sufferers)
	Photo-/phonophobia Nausea/vomiting	Classical and common migraine
	Pain increased by lying down/ bending over/coughing/exertion	Sinusitis Tumour?
	Stress	Tension headache, Migraine

Differential diagnosis

Eye strain

Eye strain can be responsible for frontal headaches. There may be occupational pointers, e.g. people using computers for long periods. Refer to an optometrist. Headache may also be a symptom of glaucoma; if suspected, refer immediately to a doctor.

Meningitis

In meningitis there may be a severe generalised headache associated with fever, nausea, neck stiffness, pain behind knees when extended (Kernig's sign) and a purpuric rash in later stages. Refer urgently any child with headache, high temperature and who is unable to bend head forward easily.

Cluster headache

This is a condition of unknown cause that predominantly affects men between the ages of 40 and 60. Typically, headaches occur at the same time each day and last for between 10 minutes and 3 hours. About half of sufferers have attacks at night. Pain is sudden in onset, intense and 'boring' and localised around one eye. The affected eye becomes red and watery and there may be nasal congestion. Attacks persist for between a few weeks and a few months, with periods of remission of months or years. Refer immediately to a doctor.

Subarachnoid haemorrhage

Subarachnoid haemorrhage is caused by bleeding between the meningeal layers covering the spinal cord. There is sudden intense severe occipital headache, often described as 'the worst I've ever had'. It is often accompanied by nausea and vomiting. There may be transient loss of consciousness. Refer urgently to Accident & Emergency.

Temporal arteritis

Temporal arteritis is inflammation of the temporal artery running down the side of the head just in front of the ear. It occurs almost exclusively in elderly people. There is severe unilateral pain, and the area of the temple is inflamed and tender to the touch. There may be associated jaw pain and generalised rheumatic pains. Refer immediately to a doctor.

Space-occupying lesions

These lesions may be caused by tumour, haematoma or abscess. The pain can be localised or diffuse. It may be initially mild and get progressively worse. It may be severe on waking in the morning and lessen after getting up. It is made worse by coughing, sneezing or lying down. Refer if suspected. Symptoms may sometimes be confused with sinusitis, but the latter is usually associated with symptoms of upper respiratory tract infection or allergic rhinitis.

Trigeminal neuralgia

Inflammation of the trigeminal nerve occurs in people mainly over the age of 50 and is more common in women than men. The pain is intensely sharp, and cutting or searing in nature. Pain is experienced in either the forehead or the side of the head, around the eye, with redness and lacrimation, the cheek and upper jaw, or the lower jaw, depending on which branch of the trigeminal nerve is affected. Refer immediately to a doctor.

Symptoms and circumstances for referral

- sudden onset and/or very severe headache
- headache after head injury
- headache of long duration
- recurring headaches (excluding diagnosed migraine)
- headaches worsening over time
- headache accompanied by nausea/vomiting (except as part of diagnosed migraine), drowsiness
- vision affected
- pupils uneven or not reacting to light
- child under 12 (urgent if with neck stiffness, fever or rash)
- cluster headache symptoms.

Treatment

This section covers oral non-prescription medicines for most types of pain, including tension headache, migraine, sinusitis, dental pain and musculoskeletal pain. Treatment for dysmenorrhoea pain is covered in Chapter 31.
Non-prescription oral analgesics are based on three compounds:

1. aspirin
2. ibuprofen
3. paracetamol.

Clinical evidence shows that all three compounds are effective analgesics and antipyretics, and that ibuprofen is generally the most effective.

Aspirin and ibuprofen

Action and uses

- Aspirin and ibuprofen are non-steroidal anti-inflammatory drugs (NSAIDs).
- NSAIDs exert their therapeutic action by blocking the enzyme cyclo-oxygenase, which prevents the formation of prostaglandins from arachidonic acid, produced when tissue is damaged; prostaglandins are major contributors to inflammation and pain. The action of NSAIDs is local at the site of inflammation.
- NSAIDs also inhibit production of cytoprotective prostaglandins in the gastric mucosa, accounting for their tendency to cause gastrointestinal irritation, although the incidence is much lower with ibuprofen than aspirin.
- Aspirin and ibuprofen are licensed for treatment of mild and moderate pain from a wide variety of causes, including dental and musculoskeletal pain and dysmenorrhoea, where their anti-inflammatory activity is particularly useful. They also have antipyretic action and are used in cold and flu medicines.

Adverse reactions, cautions and contraindications

- Aspirin and ibuprofen have similar side-effects, although side-effects are generally less pronounced with ibuprofen.
- The most common side-effects are gastric irritation and bleeding. Both drugs should be avoided by patients with ulcers or a history of gastric problems. Minor gastric side-effects can be reduced by taking the drugs with or after food.
- Hypersensitivity reactions to aspirin are much more likely to occur in patients with asthma or allergic problems than in the normal population. One in 10 patients with asthma may be hypersensitive and suffer severe bronchospasm. Other reactions are urticaria, angioedema and rhinitis. The incidence of hypersensitivity to ibuprofen is much lower than with aspirin, but the drug should be avoided by patients with asthma and individuals who are sensitive to aspirin, unless they have taken ibuprofen before without problems.
- Aspirin and ibuprofen should not be recommended to patients with renal, cardiac or hepatic disease: both medications may impair both liver and kidney function.
- Aspirin and ibuprofen should be used with caution in elderly patients, as renal function tends to decline with age and also because the elderly tend to be particularly vulnerable to gastric side-effects.

- Aspirin and ibuprofen should be avoided during pregnancy.
- Aspirin has been associated with Reye's syndrome, a rare but potentially fatal brain condition in infants and children. Aspirin is not licensed for use in children under16 years and it should also be avoided by breastfeeding women. However, there is no evidence of an association between ibuprofen and Reye's syndrome and it is licensed for sale for use in children and babies from the age of 3 months.

Interactions

- Aspirin potentiates the anticoagulant effect of warfarin and other coumarins because of its inhibitory effect on platelet aggregation and inhibition of vitamin K synthesis. Ibuprofen may also enhance the effect of anticoagulants. Patients on anticoagulant therapy should avoid over-the-counter (OTC) aspirin and ibuprofen.
- Aspirin and, to a lesser extent, ibuprofen reduce excretion of methotrexate, and can cause life-threatening rises in serum levels. Concurrent administration should therefore be avoided.
- Ibuprofen reduces the excretion of lithium and can raise plasma concentrations to toxic levels. It may also antagonise the diuretic and antihypertensive effects of diuretics, and should not be recommended to patients taking these drugs.

Paracetamol

Action and uses

The mechanism of action of paracetamol is not well understood. It has little anti-inflammatory activity but is an effective analgesic and antipyretic. It may selectively inhibit cyclo-oxygenase in the central nervous system rather than in peripheral tissues. It also appears to act peripherally at pain chemoreceptors.

Toxicity

- Paracetamol is very safe at normal therapeutic dosages; its only major drawback is hepatotoxicity in overdose.
- Paracetamol is metabolised in the liver, where it is converted to a highly toxic intermediate that is normally detoxified by conjugation with glutathione. In overdose, this detoxification mechanism is overwhelmed and the free toxic metabolite causes hepatitis and necrosis, which can prove fatal.
- Paracetamol poisoning is particularly dangerous as the toxic level may not be greatly above the therapeutic level. Also, symptoms of overdose may not appear for 2 days or more, allowing unwitting overdosage to continue.
- Fatalities have occurred in patients who were taking large doses, or two or more preparations containing paracetamol, for a minor ailment such as a cold. It is therefore extremely important to ensure that patients do not exceed the recommended dosage and do not use more than one paracetamol-containing product at a time.
- OTC pack sizes of products containing aspirin and paracetamol and the total amounts that can be supplied are restricted to reduce the incidence of poisoning (see *Medicines Ethics and Practice* for details).

Additional constituents

- Most proprietary OTC oral analgesics are not simple formulations of aspirin, ibuprofen or paracetamol, but combination products containing other analgesics and sometimes other constituents.
- The theory behind combination products is that they will be more effective than one drug used alone and that the dose of each analgesic can be reduced, lessening the possibility of adverse effects. Further additional components are sometimes included to treat symptoms associated with pain.
- Leading medical opinion (e.g. as represented in the *British National Formulary*) does not generally favour combined analgesics, claiming that low doses of additional ingredients may reduce the severity but increase the range of side-effects without producing significant extra pain relief. Clinical evidence indicates that additional constituents add little to analgesic efficacy.

Codeine and dihydrocodeine

- Codeine is combined with aspirin, paracetamol and ibuprofen in many OTC analgesic products, and also in the formulary preparations co-codamol (with paracetamol) and co-codaprin (with aspirin). Dihydrocodeine is included with paracetamol in one OTC product, and at a higher dose in co-dydramol tablets, which are prescription-only medicines (POM).
- Codeine and dihydocodeine are opioid analgesics that act directly on opiate receptors in the brain, producing analgesia, respiratory depression, euphoria and sedation. They are weak narcotic analgesics, useful for the treatment of mild to moderate pain. Their major side-effect at non-prescription dosages is constipation.

Caffeine

- Many OTC analgesics contain caffeine, the rationale being that, as a central nervous system stimulant, it will alleviate the depression often associated with pain.
- Most preparations contain low doses, although they may be sufficient to add to gastrointestinal adverse effects. Caffeine is also habit-forming and may itself induce headache in large doses or on withdrawal.

Antihistamines

Tension in muscles at the back of the neck is thought to be a contributory factor to tension headache. Sedating antihistamines are included in some products for their claimed muscle-relaxant effect.

Migraine treatments

Migraine can often be treated with paracetamol, ibuprofen or aspirin alone, or with combination products containing them. There are also some non-prescription medicines specifically licensed for the treatment of migraine. One such is a co-formulation of paracetamol, codeine and the antihistamine buclizine, included for its antiemetic action. Other specific migraine treatments are reviewed below.

Sumatriptan

- Sumatriptan is one of a group of compounds known as triptans. Triptans are $5HT_{1D}$-receptor agonists; they cause constriction of the cerebral arteries and counteract the cranial vasodilatation thought to be responsible for migraine attacks. Triptans are now established as a first-line treatment for migraine.

- Sumatriptan is licensed for pharmacy sale for acute relief of migraine attacks, with or without aura, in adults aged 18–65 years. Treatment may not be supplied for prophylaxis or for patients who:
  - are pregnant or breastfeeding
  - have existing medical conditions, including cardiovascular conditions, hypertension, peripheral vascular disease, liver or kidney disorders
  - have any neurological condition or symptoms, including epilepsy
  - are allergic to the drug
  - are taking concurrent medication for migraine
  - are assessed as having a high cardiovascular risk, using the factors in the cardiovascular risk prediction charts in the *British National Formulary*.
- The dose is one 50 mg tablet, taken as soon as possible after the onset of an attack. A second dose may be taken after 2 hours if migraine recurs. If there is no response to the first tablet, a second tablet should not be taken for the same attack. Maximum dosage is two tablets in 24 hours.
- Referral to a doctor should be made if:
  - attacks last longer than 24 hours, become more frequent or symptoms change
  - the patient generally has four or more attacks per month
  - the patient does not completely recover between attacks
  - the patient is over 50 years of age and is suffering a migraine attack for the first time.
- Side-effects are usually mild and transient.
- Sumatriptan should be avoided by patients taking selective serotonin reuptake inhibitors, monoamine oxidase inhibitors, moclobemide, St John's wort and other vasoconstrictor migraine treatments, especially ergotamine and methysergide.

Isometheptene mucate

- Isometheptene is a sympathomimetic, used in the treatment of migraine and throbbing headache for its vasoconstrictor effect. It is combined with paracetamol in one proprietary product.
- The *British National Formulary* has classified this product as 'less suitable for prescribing' and states that other more effective treatments are available.

Prochlorperazine

- Prochlorperazine is a phenothiazine derivative.
- It is widely used on prescription for the treatment of vertigo and the prevention of nausea and vomiting.
- Prochlorperazine maleate buccal tablets are licensed for the non-prescription treatment of nausea and vomiting associated with migraine.
- The licensing conditions only permit supply if migraine has already been diagnosed by a doctor, to adults of 18 years and over. It is contraindicated in pregnant and breastfeeding women, and also in patients with impaired hepatic function, narrow-angle glaucoma, prostatic hypertrophy, epilepsy or Parkinson's disease.

Dental pain
Causes

- Dental pain (toothache) has several causes. It is not a symptom of a self-limiting condition and requires referral in all cases.
- Toothache is due to inflammation of the pulp or periodontal membrane of a tooth. Both structures are well supplied with nerves, which send impulses to the cerebral cortex where pain is perceived.
- Causes of toothache include:
- dental caries (tooth decay): often as a result of poor oral hygiene and failure to have regular dental check-ups
- dental abscess: arising from an infection in decayed dental pulp
- pericornitis: infection in the soft tissue covering impacted wisdom teeth. It occurs in young adults between the ages of 18 and 25 years
- dry socket: due to poor healing and inflammation following dental extraction
- gingival recession: starting from early middle age the gums begin to recede from the base of the teeth, exposing nerves which are very sensitive to stimuli such as heat, cold or sweetness
- trigeminal neuralgia (see above): attacks can sometimes occur following dental treatment.

Signs and symptoms

- dental caries: continuous, throbbing pain
- dental abscess: severe continuous pain with localised swelling; the affected tooth may be slightly raised from its socket
- pericornitis: localised soreness in the soft tissue overlying the impacted tooth, developing into pain if not treated
- dry socket: localised continuous pain in the area of the socket
- gingival recession: localised sharp pain of short duration on exposure to heat, cold or sweet stimuli.

Symptoms and circumstances for referral

Referral is necessary in all cases, although analgesics can be recommended until a dentist or doctor can be seen.

Treatment

In theory, ibuprofen and aspirin are the most effective analgesics as they act at the site of the pain, rather than centrally, in the manner of paracetamol and opioids. But many people find that paracetamol, perhaps in combination with an opioid, is more effective for them.

Even so, OTC analgesics may provide little relief from severe dental pain. Tooth tinctures and clove oil have a counterirritant effect, producing a sensation of warmth that masks pain for a short period. However, they can cause burns to the gums if used repeatedly.

Self-assessment

Multiple choice questions

1–3. (Closed-book, classification)

Questions 1–3 concern the following headache symptoms:

a.   a throbbing headache on one side of the head
b.   a dull headache extending from the top of the head down to the muscles of the neck
c.   a headache in the forehead and around the eyes, and a blocked nose
d.   a sudden intense headache at the base of the skull
e.   a headache with neck soreness and stiffness and signs of fever

Select, from (a) to (e) above, which of the following fit the symptoms described above:

1.   Sinusitis
2.   Subdural haematoma
3.   Tension headache

4.   (Open-book, multiple completion)
     Which of the following would be POM?

a.   a pack of 32 tablets containing co-dydramol 7.46 mg and paracetamol 500 mg
b.   a pack of 48 tablets containing co-dydramol 7.46 mg and paracetamol 500 mg
c.   a pack of 16 tablets containing co-dydramol 10 mg and paracetamol 500 mg

Tips

Be sure that you are fit and ready to take an examination. If there is any circumstance that could undermine your performance such as illness or some serious personal event, do not sit the exam. In the registration examination, you are allowed to withdraw without penalty for any reason, including feeling unprepared, at any time up until entering the exam hall. However, just feeling unprepared is not an allowable reason for withdrawing from an MPharm exam.

Eye and ear

| Ear problems | 33 |
| Eye conditions | 37 |

chapter 5
Ear problems

Earache
Causes

- In adults, earache may sometimes be associated with an upper respiratory tract infection and, as long as the pain is not severe, can be treated with oral analgesics for up to 48 hours, before referral if the condition does not improve.
- Earache in children should always be referred, as otitis media (infection of the middle ear) is fairly common and repeated attacks can lead to permanent damage if not managed properly. Use of an oral analgesic can be advised until a doctor can be seen.
- Barotrauma: some people suffer severe ear pain when flying. For information on the cause and treatment, see the case study below and the answer on p. 215.

Treatment

- Oral analgesics (see Chapter 4).
- Ear drops containing choline salicylate, which has an analgesic and anti-inflammatory effect, are available without prescription but they are not generally recommended.

Ear wax
Causes

- Cerumen (ear wax) is an oily fluid produced in the ear. It combines with exfoliated skin cells to form a protective waxy layer. In some people excessively sticky cerumen is produced that cannot be removed by the normal natural processes, and a waxy plug forms that causes discomfort and can affect hearing.
- Pharmacists should not attempt to diagnose ear wax. Patients often incorrectly ascribe their ear symptoms to it, but the presence of wax can only be confirmed by examination with an auriscope. Pharmacists can, however, offer advice on cerumenolytics once the condition has been diagnosed by a doctor or suitably qualified nurse.
- Syringing is usually necessary to remove ear wax, although cerumenolytics can be used in advance to soften, loosen and partially dissolve it.

Treatment

- Several approaches are taken to loosening and dissolving wax in the ear, including the use of aqueous and oily solvents and surfactants, and oxygen generation to facilitate penetration of water into the plug. Constituents of cerumenolytic products include:

- fixed and volatile oils, as wax solvents
- glycerol, as a softener
- docusate, a surfactant facilitating the penetration of water
- urea hydrogen peroxide; this reacts with naturally produced catalase enzyme to release oxygen and help break up wax mechanically, while urea increases penetration
- paradichlorobenzene, claimed to assist penetration of oils into wax plugs.

- Little difference in efficacy has been found between cerumenolytics, and it has been reported that they are no more effective than using warm water or saline shortly before syringing.
- The *British National Formulary* recommends olive oil, almond oil or sodium bicarbonate ear drops for softening wax before syringing.

Otitis externa
Causes

Otitis externa is inflammation of the external auditory canal. The acute form is usually caused by bacterial infection, but it may also be fungal or viral. The chronic form is eczematous and may be atopic or a contact dermatitis. Dermatitis may become infected and the two types of otitis externa can exist together.

Treatment

- Mild eczematous otitis externa affecting the pinna can be treated with hydrocortisone cream (see Chapter 27).
- Aluminium acetate is astringent and hygroscopic and produces an acidic environment that is hostile to pathogenic bacteria. Aluminium Acetate (13%) Ear Drops BP can be used as an anti-inflammatory for eczematous otitis externa in the external ear canal.
- Acetic acid has antibacterial activity. A 2% spray solution of acetic acid is licensed for the treatment of superficial infections of the external auditory canal in adults and children over the age of 12 years. Use should be discontinued and medical advice sought if symptoms do not improve within 48 hours of starting treatment.

Symptoms and circumstances for referral

- Patients seeking advice on ear problems should be referred if they report any of the following:
- pain
- deafness
- vertigo
- tinnitus
- 'blocked' ears
- discharge
- foreign body in ear

- bleeding
- nausea/vomiting
- neck stiffness
- any injury.

Self-assessment

Case study

A customer who is buying his holiday requirements tells you that he is flying to his destination, but is terrified because he gets excruciating pain in his ears on the descent before landing and is virtually deaf for hours afterwards. He asks if you can suggest anything to help.

Multiple choice questions

1. (Open-book; assertion/reason)
   First statement: Ear drops containing gentamicin are never used to treat chronic otitis media.
   Second statement: The Committee on Safety of Medicines has stated that topical treatment with ototoxic antibacterials is contraindicated in the presence of a perforation of the eardrum.

2. (Closed-book; multiple completion)
   For which of the following should a patient asking for treatment for an ear problem be referred to a doctor without asking any further questions?
   a. Dizziness
   b. Ringing in the ears
   c. An eczematous rash on the earlobe, caused by wearing costume jewellery earrings

3–5. (Open-book; classification)
   Questions relate to the following treatments for ear problems.
   a. Aluminium acetate 8% ear drops
   b. Audax ear drops
   c. Cerumol ear drops
   d. Molcer ear drops
   e. Sodium bicarbonate ear drops

   Which, from (a) to (e) above:
3. is not prescribable under the NHS?
4. must be freshly prepared?
5. is for the treatment of earache?

Tips

Read multiple choice questions thoroughly and make sure you understand them before answering, particularly if your first language is not English. In particular, watch out for negative expressions, such as 'not' and 'cannot', although in the registration exam these are usually highlighted to help you.

chapter 6
Eye conditions

Conditions of the cornea
Causes

There are some minor conditions of the cornea for which pharmacists can offer advice and treatment. These are:

- allergic conjunctivitis (see Chapter 23)
- infective conjunctivitis, caused by:
- viruses (mainly adenovirus or picornavirus)
- bacteria (usually *Streptococcus* or *Haemophilus*).
- subconjunctival haemorrhage, caused by rupture of a conjunctival capillary causing spread of blood over the cornea. It looks alarming but it is painless, vision is not affected and it is usually of no significance. There is no treatment and the blood cannot be washed out of the eye
- dacrocystitis: the lacrimal sac, which drains tears into the nasolacrimal duct in the corner of the eye, becomes blocked or in young children may not open, and tears overflow. It may be cleared by gentle massage in the inner corner of eye, but if it does not clear, the patient should be referred.

Signs and symptoms

The features of minor corneal conditions are set out in Table 6.1.

Table 6.1 Signs and symptoms of minor eye conditions

Feature	Significance	Possible indication
Eyes affected	Both	Viral or allergic conjunctivitis
	Both, but one before the other	Bacterial conjunctivitis
Discharge	Watery	Viral or allergic conjunctivitis
	Purulent	Bacterial conjunctivitis
Pain/discomfort	No pain	All conjunctivitis Subconjunctival haemorrhage
	Itching/gritty	Bacterial or viral conjunctivitis
	Itching only Pain	Allergic conjunctivitis More serious conditions
Redness	Generalised, diffuse	All conjunctivitis
	Around centre of eye	More serious conditions

(continued)

Table 6.1 (cont.)

	Localised areas of sclera	More serious conditions
Duration	2–3 days	Infective conjunctivitis
	Variable, depending on exposure to allergen	Allergic conjunctivitis
	Up to 10 days	Subconjunctival haemorrhage
	> 1 week	More serious conditions
Associated factors	None	Bacterial
	Cough and cold symptoms	Viral
	Allergic rhinitis symptoms	Allergic conjunctivitis

Differential diagnosis

Glaucoma

- Open-angle (chronic) glaucoma results from an increase in ocular pressure due to an imbalance between production and drainage of aqueous humour. It develops slowly and initially is symptomless, but eventually it produces headache and loss of visual field. It affects both eyes and can cause blindness if not treated.
- Closed-angle (acute) glaucoma is due to obstruction to drainage of aqueous humour. It presents as severe pain in one eye, accompanied by headache, nausea and vomiting. Visual field is reduced and haloes may be seen around lights.

Episcleritis

In episcleritis there is inflammation of the sclera, the tissue immediately beneath the conjunctiva, producing a localised patch of redness. It is usually painless or there may be a dull ache. It is most common in young women. It is self-limiting, but could take several weeks to resolve.

Scleritis

Scleritis is of similar appearance to episcleritis but much more painful. It is often associated with autoimmune conditions such as rheumatoid arthritis.

Uveitis (iritis)

Uveitis is inflammation of the uveal tract (the structures around the iris). There is localised central redness, with pain and photophobia, and vision may be impaired. It may be associated with rheumatoid arthritis or ulcerative colitis.

Keratitis (corneal ulcer)

Inflammation of the cornea is keratitis. There is severe pain with a watery discharge and photophobia. Redness is concentrated in the centre of the eye. It may result from trauma, long-term use of steroid eye drops or use of soft contact lenses.

Dry eye

Dry eye is a chronic condition, often associated with a systemic disorder such as rheumatoid arthritis. It may cause irritation and photophobia.

Symptoms and circumstances for referral

- pain in the eye, as distinct from superficial soreness, grittiness or itchiness
- redness localised to one area of the eye surface
- disturbance of vision
- pupils of abnormal shape or uneven pupils
- pupils reacting unevenly to light
- eye symptoms with headache and/or nausea/vomiting
- recurrent subconjunctival haemorrhage
- dry eyes.

Essential criteria for distinguishing between minor and potentially more serious eye conditions are set out in Table 6.2.

Table 6.2 Distinguishing criteria between minor and potentially more serious eye conditions

Minor eye conditions	Potentially more serious eye conditions
Irritation and discomfort, but no pain	Pain
Redness over entire eye surface	Localised redness
Vision unaffected (although there may be slight blurring)	Vision affected

Treatment

Allergic conjunctivitis

See Chapter 23.

Infective conjunctivitis

- Bacteria and viruses are both causes of infective conjunctivitis and it may be clinically difficult to distinguish between them. Over-the-counter treatment of any superficial infective conjunctivitis with an antibacterial agent is considered appropriate, as it may help prevent secondary bacterial infection.
- Non-prescription antimicrobial compounds available for the treatment of these infections are:
- chloramphenicol
- propamidine and dibromopropamidine isetionates.

Chloramphenicol

- Chloramphenicol is active against a wide range of ocular pathogens. It has been the first-choice prescription antibiotic for minor eye infections for many years, and chloramphenicol eye drops were reclassified for pharmacy sale in 2005 for use for adults and children aged 2 years and over.

- Dosage is one drop into the infected eye every 2 hours for the first 48 hours and then every 4 hours, during waking hours only. Treatment should be continued for 5 days, if symptoms improve.
- Chloramphenicol eye drops should not be used in patients hypersensitive to chloramphenicol, who have experienced myelosuppression during previous exposure to chloramphenicol or with a family history of blood dyscrasias, and it is not recommended for pregnant or breastfeeding women.
- Prolonged or frequent intermittent use should be avoided, as it may increase the likelihood of sensitisation and emergence of resistant organisms.
- The drops should not be used for more than 5 days, and patients should be referred if symptoms do not improve within 48 hours of starting treatment.
- As with all ocular antibiotic and most other eye preparations, contact lenses should not be worn during treatment and soft contact lenses should not be replaced for 24 hours after completing treatment.
- In the pharmacy, chloramphenicol eye drops should be stored in a refrigerator at 2–8°C. Once opened, the drops should be discarded after 5 days.
- In June 2007, chloramphenicol eye ointment was reclassified from prescription only (POM) to pharmacy sale (P) for the treatment of acute bacterial conjunctivitis.

Propamidine and dibromopropamidine isetionates

- Propamidine and dibromopropamidine isetionates are aromatic diamidine antiseptics. They have been used for the treatment of bacterial conjunctivitis for more than 60 years and have always been available without prescription, but chloramphenicol is considered the drug of choice and the *British National Formulary* regards propamidine and dibromopropamidine as of little value.
- Eye drops are formulated with propamidine isetionate 0.1% and eye ointment with dibromopropamidine isetionate 0.15%. Both can be used for adults and children.
- The ointment persists longer on the corneal surface and needs to be applied only twice daily, but can cause stickiness and blurring of vision. Drops are used four times daily. Treatment should be continued for 24 hours after symptoms have cleared. If symptoms do not significantly improve within 48 hours, treatment should be discontinued and the patient referred for medical advice.
- Both products should be stored at room temperature and discarded not more than 1 month after opening.

Conditions of the eyelid

- There is one minor condition – stye (hordeolum) – for which pharmacists can offer advice and treatment. It is caused by staphylococcal infection of a hair follicle at the base of an eyelash.
- Principal symptoms are pain, redness, swelling and irritation. Initially, the whole of the lid may be affected, then swelling becomes localised, and a yellow pustule may develop near the lid margin.
- Treatment is with dibromopropanidine isetionate ointment.

Differential diagnosis and factors for referral

Referral should be made if any of the conditions described below are suspected.

Blepharitis

Blepharitis is chronic inflammation of the lid margins, affecting both eyes. There are three main types: staphylococcal, seborrhoeic (frequently associated with seborrhoea of the scalp, eyebrows and ears) and contact dermatitis (due to cosmetics). The lid margins appear raw and red, with irritation, burning and itching. If contact dermatitis is the cause then there is generally a history of atopy, and other areas of skin may be affected. Scales are frequently seen on the lashes of both upper and lower lids, which tend to be dry in staphylococcal infections and greasy in seborrhoeic blepharitis. The lids become deformed in staphylococcal blepharitis due to ulceration. Lashes are frequently lost or may be distorted, turn inwards and rub on the cornea; this in turn can cause conjunctivitis. Mild seborrhoeic blepharitis can often be managed with eyelid hygiene without prescribed medication. However, medical diagnosis is always necessary first and the condition may not respond to over-the-counter treatment.

Chalazion (meibomian cyst)

A chalazion is a cyst of a meibomian gland: the meibomian gland secretes fluid to stop the eyelashes sticking together. It may become infected or develop into a sterile chronic granuloma, a firm, painless lump in the lid which gradually enlarges. Initially, the chalazion may resemble a stye but is not inflamed. Chalazia usually grow inwards towards the conjunctival surface, which may be slightly reddened or elevated. Infected cysts are treated as styes. A third of cases will resolve spontaneously and virtually all will resorb within 2 years, but they are often surgically removed before then.

Ectropion

This is mainly a condition of old age, as is entropion (see below). Sagging and turning outward of the lower eyelid occur from a natural loss of muscle tone and orbital fat. Tears overflow and there is insufficient lubrication and protection for the eye. The lower lid may become chronically infected and scarred. This then requires surgical correction.

Entropion

The lower lids turn inwards and lid margins and eyelashes abrade the surface of the eye. Lashes may fall out and susceptibility to infection is increased. Entropion requires surgical correction.

Basal cell carcinoma

Basal cell carcinoma presents as a reddish nodule on the eyelid. There is no pain or discomfort. There may be a history of prolonged exposure to sun or ultraviolet light.

Other eye problems

Sore and 'tired' eyes

- Redness and mild irritation in the eyes can be caused by activities such as driving and close work, and environmental pollutants, including tobacco smoke.
- Several eye drop preparations, based mainly on astringents and vasoconstrictors, are available without prescription:
  - Several products contain distilled witch hazel (hamamelis water), obtained from the bark of a shrub, with astringent and anti-inflammatory properties.
  - Naphazoline, a sympathomimetic vasoconstrictor, is included in some ophthalmic preparations to shrink the dilated blood vessels that cause redness.

Dry eyes

- Dry eye (keratoconjunctivitis sicca) is a chronic condition characterised by dryness of the surface of the eye. It is caused by either a deficiency of conjunctival mucus, due to the absence or significant impairment of the mucin-producing goblet cells of the conjunctiva, or tear deficiency, the latter often associated with rheumatoid arthritis.
- The cause of dry eye requires medical diagnosis.
- Treatment is usually with tear substitutes ('artificial tears'), containing compounds that enhance wetting, viscosity and stability of tears. These are: hypromellose, polyvinyl alcohol (PVA), carbomer 940, and hydrophobic ocular lubricants containing liquid and soft paraffins, such as Simple Eye Ointment. All preparations are available as P medicines.

Self-assessment

Case study

A man asks for your advice about his eye. He tells you that he had a stye a couple of months ago, but it had cleared up after a few days following treatment with an over-the-counter eye ointment he had bought in another pharmacy. However, a little lump has now formed on his eyelid where the stye was. It doesn't hurt at all, but it is a bit of a nuisance and he wonders if you can suggest anything to get rid of it. Can you?

Multiple choice questions

1. (Closed-book, multiple completion)
   Which of the following signs and symptoms, in an adult patient asking for advice about her eyes, would lead you to make immediate referral to a doctor?
   a. pain and redness around the centre of one eye; can't see properly out of it
   b. one eye completely covered in a red film of blood; no pain or discomfort; no impairment of vision
   c. both eyes slightly red across the entire surface; feeling of soreness and itchiness; slight discharge leaving a yellowish crust around the eyelids when it dries; no pain; no impairment of vision.

2–4.(Open-book, classification)

   Questions 2–4 concern the ophthalmic preparations listed below:

a.   Acular 0.5% eye drops

b.   Artelac SDU

c.   Isopto Plain eye drops

d.   Voltarol Ophtha eye drops

e.   Zinc sulphate 0.25% eye drops

   Which, from (a) to (e) above:

2.   is indicated for the treatment of hayfever?

3.   is now little used?

4.   is a POM?

5.   (Closed-book, simple completion)

   Which one of the following is not indicated for dry eye conditions?

a.   Carmellose 1% eye drops

b.   Chloramphenicol 0.5% eye drops

c.   Hydroxyethylcellulose 0.44% eye drops

d.   Polyvinyl alcohol 1.4% eye drops

e.   Povidone 5% eye drops

Tips

If you suffer from a chronic condition, e.g. migraine, and have an attack that you think has seriously adversely affected your performance during the registration exam, you can ask for your entry to be considered null and void. If granted, your mark in the exam will not be considered by the examiners (even if you have passed) and you will be treated as if you had not sat it. You will, of course, have to sit it again. In order to get consideration for your request, you will need to report your indisposition to an invigilator on the day and provide confirmation from a medical practitioner that you suffer chronically from the condition and had a severe attack during the exam.

Foot conditions

Athlete's foot   47
Foot (podiatric) problems   53
Fungal nail infection (onychomycosis)   57
Verrucas (plantar warts)
    and warts (common warts)   61

chapter 7
Athlete's foot

Tinea pedis (athlete's foot) is a topical fungal infection of the spaces between the toes.

Causes

- Athlete's foot is the commonest of a group of topical fungal infections (see Chapter 28) caused by dermatophytes, organisms that invade and proliferate on the outermost horny layer (stratum corneum) of the skin, hair and nails. They do not normally penetrate deeper into the skin or tissues. Dermatophytes tend to thrive in areas of the body that are occluded and moist.
- The common infecting organisms are *Trichophyton*, *Microsporum* and *Epidermophyton* species.
- The infection is easily transmitted in moist or humid locations, e.g. sports clubs, gyms and swimming-pool changing rooms, hence the common name of the condition. It is also associated with the use of occlusive footwear such as trainers.

Epidemiology

- Tinea pedis mainly occurs in adolescents and young adults, and is more common in males.
- It is more common in the summer months.

Signs and symptoms

- Infection usually starts in the toe webs, especially in the fourth web space (next to the little toe), where the tissue can become macerated, white and cracked.
- Infection can spread to the soles, heels and borders of the foot.
- Painful itching is common.
- The skin may fissure and allow entry of bacterial infection.
- The sole may be affected, making the condition more difficult to diagnose and differentiate from psoriasis or eczema.
- With persistent infection the toenails may become involved, becoming dull, opaque and yellow in appearance. Over time the nail hardens and then starts to crumble (see Chapter 8).

Differential diagnosis

- Eczema: an inflammatory skin condition characterised by areas of redness, itching and weeping, which can become scaly, crusty and hardened. The condition may be endogenous or caused by an irritant or allergen in contact with the skin.
- Psoriasis: a chronic skin condition characterised by well-defined red patches covered with white scales.
- Erythrasma, a bacterial infection: the usual mild form responds to azole antifungals (see below).

Circumstances for referral

- severe infection spreading beyond the toe spaces on to the sole or upper surface of the foot, or to the toenails
- signs of secondary bacterial infection
- infection unresponsive to antifungal topical treatment
- diabetic patients (diabetic patients with any foot problems should always be referred to a chiropodist or doctor: see Chapter 8)
- suspected eczema or psoriasis.

Treatment

- Treatments available for the treatment of athlete's foot are antifungals. Salicylic acid is also included in some preparations.
- Terbinafine and the imidazoles are widely accepted as being the most effective treatments for athlete's foot. Little overall difference in efficacy has been found between them, although terbinafine clears infections up to four times more quickly. Griseofulvin has also been found an effective treatment.
- Undecenoic acid and its derivatives are thought to be suitable for mild forms of athlete's foot characterised by dry scaling of tissue, but are less effective where the skin is macerated and moist. Undecenoic acid and tolnaftate have been found to be about equally effective.
- Some over-the-counter creams containing an imidazole and hydrocortisone are licensed for the treatment of athlete's foot and associated inflammation and irritation.

Antifungals
Compounds available are: imidazoles, terbinafine, griseofulvin, tolnaftate, undecenoates and benzoic acid.

Imidazoles
- Imidazoles licensed for treatment of athlete's foot without prescription are clotrimazole, econazole, ketoconazole, miconazole and sulconazole.
- They act by inhibiting the biosynthesis of ergosterol, a constituent of the fungal cell membrane, resulting in disruption of the cell.

- These compounds also possess activity against Gram-positive bacteria, which is useful, as secondary bacterial infection may complicate the fungal infection.
- Application twice or three times daily is recommended, and treatment for at least a month is generally advised to ensure that this tenacious infection is eradicated.

Terbinafine
- Terbinafine is an allylamine derivative with a broad spectrum of antifungal activity.
- It is available as a 1% cream which is applied once or twice daily for 1 week, a 1% gel which is used once daily for 1 week, and a cutaneous solution which requires only a single application.

Griseofulvin
- Griseofulvin is exclusively active against dermatophytes, through inhibition of cellular mitosis. It also binds to host cell keratin and reduces its degradation by fungal keratinases. It may also interfere with dermatophyte DNA production.
- It is available as a 1% topical spray. One spray is applied daily, increasing to three sprays daily for more severe or extensive infection affecting the sides or soles of the feet. Treatment should be continued for 10 days after lesions have disappeared. The treatment period should not exceed 4 weeks.

Tolnaftate
- Tolnaftate is believed to act by distorting fungal hyphae and stunting mycelial growth. It is active against all species responsible for athlete's foot but has no antibacterial activity.
- It should be used twice daily and treatment should be continued for up to 6 weeks. It is well tolerated when applied to intact or broken skin, although slight stinging on application is probable. Skin reactions are rare and include irritation and contact dermatitis.

Undecenoates
- Both undecenoic acid and zinc undecenoate are used in proprietary athlete's foot preparations.
- Zinc undecenoate has astringent properties, which helps to reduce the irritation and inflammation caused by the infection.
- Undecenoic acid, the active antifungal entity, is liberated from the zinc salt on contact with moisture on the skin.
- Up to 4 weeks' treatment may be needed to produce therapeutic results. Irritation occurs rarely after application of undecenoic acid or its salts.

Benzoic acid
- Benzoic acid has antifungal activity, lowering the intracellular pH of infecting organisms.
- It is combined with salicylic acid (see below) in an emulsifying ointment

base in Benzoic Acid Ointment Compound BP (Whitfield's ointment). This preparation has been in use for over 90 years but more cosmetically acceptable products are now available.

■ Benzoic acid may cause irritation of the skin, and should not come into contact with the eyes or mucous membranes.

Salicylic acid

■ Salicylic acid alone has little or no antifungal activity but it facilitates the penetration of other drugs into the epidermis. Preparations for athlete's foot containing salicylic acid therefore also contain antifungal constituents; it is present in Whitfield's ointment and some proprietary preparations.

■ At concentrations above 2% salicylic acid has a keratolytic effect, causing the keratin layer of the skin to shed. Keratolysis is achieved by increasing the hydration of the stratum corneum, softening the cells and facilitating dissolution of the intracellular cement that bonds the cells together so that they separate and detach (desquamate). Moisture is essential to this process and is provided by either the water in the formulation or the occlusive effect produced by its application to the skin.

■ Although salicylic acid is readily absorbed through the skin, salicylate poisoning is highly unlikely to result from application to a small area for the limited period of treatment for athlete's foot.

Additional advice

■ Wash and thoroughly dry feet and toes daily, particularly between the toes.
■ Do not share towels in communal changing rooms.
■ Wash towels frequently.
■ Change socks daily.
■ Wear flip-flops or plastic sandals in communal changing rooms and showers.
■ When at home leave shoes and socks off as much as possible.

Self-assessment

Case study

A young man, who is a keen footballer, tells you he has tried several different treatments for athlete's foot, but although they clear the condition up the infection keeps coming back. He wants you to recommend something that will really get rid of it this time. What would be your recommendation and advice?

Multiple choice questions

1. (Closed-book, assertion/reason)
   First statement: Salicylic acid is of no use in the treatment of athlete's foot.
   Second statement: Salicylic acid has little or no antifungal activity.

2-4. (Open-book, classification)

Questions 2–4 concern the following treatments for athlete's foot:

a.   benzoic acid

b.   clotrimazole

c.   griseofulvin

d.   terbinafine

e.   undecenoic acid

Which of the above:

2.   is only available as a spray?

3.   has a maximum recommended treatment duration of 4 weeks?

4.   is a constituent of Whitfield's ointment?

Tips

In examinations, do not waste your own and the marker's time by providing an irrelevant answer ('waffle') to a question if you do not know the correct answer. It will get you no marks.

chapter 8
Foot (podiatric) problems

Hard and soft corns and calluses
Causes

- Corns and calluses are variously known as hyperkeratosis, clavus, heloma and tyloma, but all essentially describe the same condition – a local thickening of the epidermis as a result of intermittent pressure meeting with constant resistance over some bony prominence on the foot.
- The irritation caused by this rubbing increases the blood supply, bringing extra nutrition to the basal layers of the epidermis, resulting in increased proliferation of cells and thickened areas of hard, insoluble mass. Pressure on nerve endings in the dermis causes pain.
- Hard corns form on the outer aspects of the toes as a result of rubbing against shoes.
- Soft corns usually occur between the toes and are softened by the presence of moisture (sweat).
- Calluses are more diffuse areas of thickening on the sole or the side of the foot.
- Contributory factors to these conditions include:
- ill-fitting footwear
- foot deformities
- occupational – workers who spend a lot of time on their feet or walking
- obesity.

Signs and symptoms

Hard corns
- soreness, which becomes a burning or throbbing pain on walking or standing
- a thick, rounded, yellowish mass, which may be surrounded by an area of inflammation, with a round or crescent-shaped nucleus varying in size from a pinhead to a lentil
- occur on dorsal surfaces over joints, under the ends of toes, beside nails, between toes and under the nail at the ends of toes.

Soft corns
- soreness and pain and the feeling of a foreign body between the toes
- a white, soft rubbery mass between the toes
- tissue may be thin and peel off easily to expose bright pink tissue beneath, with a nucleus conforming to the underlying bone.

Calluses
- pain and burning sensation, and possibly a feeling of skin 'tightness'
- a creamy yellow mass that feels hard, with no nucleus.

Symptoms and circumstances for referral

- Particular care is needed with certain groups of at-risk patients wanting to self-care for foot problems, including elderly people and patients with diabetes or peripheral vascular disease. These patients should be referred to either a chiropodist or their general practitioner, for the following reasons:
- Patients with diabetes often have poor peripheral circulation, are more liable to ischaemic foot lesions than healthy people and will recover less readily from any minor foot damage. In addition, peripheral neuropathy may result in a decreased perception of pain so that any injury to the feet may not be noticed.
- Vision may also be impaired, particularly in elderly patients with diabetes, making it more difficult to see any damage that may have occurred.
- Elderly people often do not have the physical mobility or the dexterity to manage their own treatment properly.

Treatment

Epidermabrasion
- Epidermabrasion is a physical process that removes horny skin using a mechanical aid. Several gently abrasive materials and appliances are available, including emery boards, foot files, pumice stones and synthetic pumice-like blocks.
- Careful technique is important for the safe and successful removal of corns and calluses, using the following procedure:
- To soften the skin, soak the foot in mild soapy water for a few minutes or apply a moisturising or softening cream.
- Rub soap on to the appliance and gently rub the corn or callus for 5 minutes.
- Repeat the process nightly for 1 week, then review. There is no need to remove the hard skin completely, just enough to relieve pain or irritation.
- Avoid ill-fitting shoes to help prevent recurrence.

Hydrocolloid and hydrogel plasters
- Hydrocolloids and hydrogels are complex polymer formulations used in wound management. They swell in the presence of moisture absorbed from the skin.
- In corn and callus plasters the hydrocolloid or hydrogel forms a soft, protective gel-like cushion that rehydrates and softens the hardened tissue. The plaster is left in place for about a week, and the corn or callused skin should come away when the plaster is removed.

Salicylic acid
- The function of salicylic acid in treating corns and calluses is to remove a thick layer of cornified skin cells, mainly through loosening the attachment of the hardened skin to the normal skin.

- The concentration in preparations ranges from about 11 to 50%.
- Corn and callus caps and plasters contain high concentrations (usually 40%) in a semisolid base spread on to a suitable backing material, contained within a ring that is either self-adhesive or attached to an adhesive plaster. They should be changed every 1–2 days for about a week, after which the callosity should lift away easily.
- An ointment containing 50% salicylic acid is also available; it should be applied nightly for 4 nights.
- Paints and liquids contain 11–17% salicylic acid, often in a collodion-based vehicle. Collodions contain pyroxylin, a nitrocellulose derivative, dissolved in a volatile solvent such as ether, acetone or alcohol. On application, the solvent evaporates, leaving on the skin an adherent, flexible, water-repellent film containing the medicament. This has the advantage of maintaining the salicylic acid at the site of application and also assists skin maceration by preventing moisture evaporation. Liquid preparations are usually applied daily for several days until the corn or callus can be easily removed.
- As salicylic acid is caustic to normal skin, care should be taken to prevent preparations from spreading beyond affected areas.
- Preparations containing high concentrations of salicylic acid should be avoided by people sensitive to aspirin.

Bunions
Causes

- A bunion is an enlargement of the first metatarsal phalangeal joint on the outside of the large toe. The deviation of the joint is known as hallux valgus.
- The cause is usually footwear that is too tight with inadequate arch support, and the regular wearing of high heels.

Signs and symptoms

- A bunion is initially painless, becoming painful as the toe displacement increases. There may be redness and some swelling.
- Motion of the joint may be restricted or painful.
- Hard corns, soft corns and calluses may develop on and between the large and second toe as a result of pressure from shoes.

Symptoms and circumstances for referral

- Referral is always necessary, for orthotic treatment (support or bracing to correct the deformity) or corrective surgery.

Treatment

- In the early stages, use of cushioning products to reduce pressure and wearing of comfortable, well-fitting shoes may slow or halt progress but cannot reverse it.

Ingrown toenail
Causes

- The main cause is poor cutting of the nail. Creating sharp corners, trimming too closely to the skin, or leaving outer edges with a ragged finish can allow the nail to grow into the skin, setting up soreness and inflammation (paronychia) which may then become infected.

Symptoms and signs

- There may be pain with spreading soreness and redness, and possible bleeding.
- Pustules may develop if infection is present.

Symptoms and circumstances for referral

- Referral is always necessary.

Self-assessment

Case study

A young woman is referred to you by your medicines counter assistant. The assistant says that she saw the woman looking at self-service foot treatments and when the assistant asked if she could help, the woman said she was looking for something to treat a callus for her grandmother. In response to your questions, the woman tells you that her grandmother is 76 years old and is a non-insulin-dependent diabetic. What would your advice be?

Multiple choice questions

1. (Open-book, simple completion)
   Which one of the following is not prescribable on the NHS for the treatment of corns?
   a. Self-adhesive corn rings 5 mm thickness
   b. Cuplex gel
   c. Duofilm paint
   d. Salactol paint
   e. Salatac gel

2. (Open-book, assertion/reason)
   First statement: Cryotherapy is the first-choice treatment for removal of corns and calluses.
   Second statement: Salicylic acid is not considered suitable for the treatment of corns and calluses.

Tips

In the registration examination, leave enough time at the end to transfer your answers to the answer sheet. You will not be allowed any extra time to do this.

chapter 9
Fungal nail infection (onychomycosis)

Causes

- Onychomycosis is infection of the nails of the fingers or toes caused by dermatophytes (fungi that live on the outer keratinous layer of the skin), yeasts or moulds.
- 90% of toenail and 50% of fingernail infections are caused by the same *Trichophyton* and *Epidermophyton* species that cause athlete's foot.
- Predisposing factors include: increasing age, male gender, diabetes, nail trauma, excessive sweating, peripheral vascular disease, poor hygiene, athlete's foot, immunodeficiency and chronic exposure of the nails to water.

Epidemiology

- Onychomycosis accounts for one-third of all fungal skin infections.
- Prevalence in adults is estimated at between 3 and 8% and there are more than 1 million sufferers in the UK.
- Infection rates in children are about 30 times lower than in adults, and in patients with diabetes about three times higher. Immunosuppressed and immunocompromised individuals also have a high susceptibility to infection.
- The main form of fungal nail infection is distal and lateral subungual onychomycosis (DLSO). It is 20–30 times more common on toenails than fingernails.

Signs and symptoms

- The nail is thickened and has turned yellow or white.
- Changes usually start at the top of the nail but may spread across to the sides and down towards the nail base.
- Debris created as a result of the infection accumulates under the nail.
- There is scaling and distortion of the nail.
- The nail may become brittle and some or all of it may break off.

Differential diagnosis

- Psoriasis of the nails may appear similar to DLSO but it is also usually present at other skin sites. There is usually fine pitting on the nail surface, small salmon-coloured 'oil drops', and fingernails on both hands are affected.

- Lichen planus is an inflammatory skin condition, the main features of which are itchy, flat-topped papules, usually on the inner surfaces of the wrists and the lower legs. Nail involvement occurs in about 10% of patients (usually in more serious cases) and fine ridging or grooving can be seen, with severe dystrophy or even complete destruction of the nail bed.
- Contact dermatitis occasionally resembles onychomycosis. Asking the patient about contact with possible irritants and finding the presence of contact dermatitis elsewhere on the body should differentiate the condition from DLSO.
- Nail trauma: repeated damage to the nail can cause distal onycholysis (loosening of the nail, starting at the free edge and spreading to the root). This leads to colonisation by microorganisms and pigmentation of the area. If the onycholytic nail is clipped and the nail bed examined, it will appear normal with no subungual debris.
- Yellow-nail syndrome is characterised by yellow nails and is commonly associated with lung disorders. The nails lack a cuticle, grow slowly and are loose or detached. All nails are affected.

Symptoms and circumstances for referral

- Patients:
- with conditions that predispose to fungal infections (e.g. immunosuppression, diabetes, peripheral circulatory disorders)
- under 18 years of age
- with nail conditions other than clearly identified DLSO
- with more than two infected nails
- with nail dystrophy or a destroyed nail
- showing no improvement after 3 months' treatment.
- Pregnant or breastfeeding women.

Treatment

- Onychomycosis is one of the most difficult fungal infections to treat because of the time it takes for the nail to grow, the hardness of the nail plate and location of the infectious process (between the nail bed and plate).

Prescription treatments
- Oral therapies. Terbinafine and itraconazole are considered the systemic treatments of choice.
- Tioconazole 28% cutaneous solution is licensed for topical treatment of onychomycosis, but there is little clinical evidence of its effectiveness.

Non-prescription treatment: amorolfine 5% nail lacquer
- Amorolfine 5% nail lacquer is licensed for pharmacy sale for the treatment of mild cases of DLSO, affecting up to two nails, in patients aged 18 years or over.

- Amorolfine is a morpholine derivative, used topically as an antifungal, with a broad spectrum of activity against dermatophytes, other fungi and yeasts. Its fungicidal action is based on ergosterol depletion and the accumulation of ignosterol in fungal cytoplasmic membrane, which causes the fungal cell wall to thicken and chitin to be deposited.
- The nail lacquer formulation builds a non-water-soluble film on the nail plate that remains at the application site for a week, acting as a depot for the drug.
- The product must be used weekly for up to 9 months, until all the infected nail has grown out and been replaced by healthy nail tissue.
- A clinical trial demonstrated an overall cure in nearly 50% of patients after weekly treatment for 6 months, with overall improvement in a further 25%.
- Adverse effects are rare and minor, amorolfine is not systematically absorbed and there are no known interactions with other drugs.

Additional advice

- A cure cannot be achieved overnight. It is important that treatment is continued and directions are followed.
- Wash and thoroughly dry feet every day.
- To prevent the infection spreading to other toes, avoid tight-fitting or occlusive shoes.
- Rest shoes periodically to limit exposure to infectious fungi.
- Use antifungal powders once a week to help keep shoes free from pathogens.
- Exercise good nail care and be alert for infection recurrence.
- Visit a podiatrist regularly.
- Infection can be passed to others through contamination of shared facilities, so do not go barefoot in the family bathroom or public places.

Self-assessment

Case study

An elderly customer reminds you that she has tried several over-the-counter products over the past 2 years for the fungal nail infection on two of her toes, but nothing has worked. She has also asked her general practitioner for treatment, but he has been reluctant to prescribe her oral antifungals because of the risk of side-effects. She says she has come back to you because she has seen something new advertised and would like to try it, but it is very expensive and she cannot afford to buy it. She wonders if there is any way that you can help her.

What is this 'new' product and how can you help her? (Note: this scenario took place in July 2006.)

Multiple choice question

1. (Open-book, assertion/reason)

    First statement: Curanail (P version of amorolfine 5% nail lacquer) is not prescribable on the NHS.

    Second statement: Curanail is not listed in the *British National Formulary*.

Tips

Boost your confidence for exams by 'positive imaging' (imagining that you have passed) and by practising self-talk and affirmations – provided that you have done the necessary study and revision.

chapter 10

Verrucas (plantar warts) and warts (common warts)

Causes

- Verrucas and warts are horny projections of skin, usually on the hands and feet, caused by the human papillomavirus (HPV).
- HPV infection is very contagious; infection is easily spread from one site to another on an infected person, and from one person to another.

Epidemiology

- Warts and verrucas are rare in children under 3 years of age. Incidence is 5–10% of children between 4 and 6 years, rising to 15–20% of young people between 16 and 18, and falling significantly in adulthood.
- Immunocompromised and immunosuppressed patients are particularly susceptible to warts and verrucas. There is also a high incidence of warts on the hands in people who handle fish or meat in their work.
- Untreated, half of warts and verrucas clear in 1 year and two-thirds in 2 years, but they are usually treated to get rid of them faster.

Signs and symptoms

Common warts

- Common warts are usually found on the hands, fingers and elbows, and on the knees in children under 12, but can occur anywhere on the body.
- In appearance, they are rough, scaly, pink or skin-coloured papules with a papillomatous rough surface; usually of less than 1 cm diameter, but can be larger; and occur singly or in groups.
- They are normally painless.

Verrucas

- Verrucas occur on the plantar surface (sole) of the foot and are painful because of downward pressure on nerve endings in the skin.
- Verrucas most commonly occur where the ball of the foot is exposed to pressure.
- They are often sore to touch and to stand or walk on.
- They appear as areas of flat, thickened skin with a harder edge around a softer centre and may be confused with plantar callus.

- On closer examination, or rubbing away the surface with a file or emery board, small black spots (telangiectasia, the ends of broken blood capillaries) can be seen.
- Occasionally, several verrucas appear together and coalesce to form a single large plaque known as a mosaic wart.

Differential diagnosis

Common warts
- Seborrhoeic warts: similar in appearance to common warts but brown in colour, and occurring mainly on the back and chest. They are benign and occur increasingly with increasing age.
- Skin tags: benign, flesh-coloured or dark brown, flat or stalk-like papillomas, occurring mainly on the neck.
- Basal and squamous cell carcinomas: malignant growths with a wart-like appearance in the early stages, usually occurring in areas of skin exposed to the sun. Referral is necessary if suspected.

Verrucas
- Plantar callus (see above and p.54).

Treatment

Treatment is the same for both verrucas and warts, and is by gradual removal of the hyperkeratotic skin layers and the viral core by keratolytic agents.

Salicylic acid
- In the treatment of warts and verrucas, salicylic acid reduces viral numbers by mechanical removal of infected tissue.
- It also stimulates production of protective antibodies in response to the mildly irritant effect of the acid.
- Some products containing salicylic acid, including ointments and collodion-based preparations, are the same as those marketed for corns and calluses.

Lactic acid
- Lactic acid is included with salicylic acid in several verruca products.
- It is corrosive and is claimed to enhance the effects of salicylic acid.
- Care must be taken that preparations do not spread on to unaffected skin.

Podophyllum resin (podophyllin)
- Podophyllum resin is obtained from the dried rhizome of the May-apple (*Podophyllum peltatum*).
- It has a potent corrosive action, and for non-prescription use it is only indicated for verrucas.
- It is cytotoxic, caustic and a powerful skin irritant; care must be taken to confine its application to the verruca.

■ There have been reports of teratogenicity and it is contraindicated in pregnancy.

Formaldehyde and glutaraldehyde
■ Formaldehyde and glutaraldehyde have antiviral activity and a direct anhidrotic effect, drying the verruca and surrounding skin.
■ Formaldehyde (0.75%) is available as an aqueous gel, and a 3% solution can be used for daily foot soaks for mosaic warts, although care must be taken to protect unaffected skin.
■ Glutaraldehyde has similar properties but appears to have no advantage over formaldehyde and may be a more potent skin sensitiser. It also stains skin brown, but this fades once treatment is discontinued.

Method of use of verruca and wart treatments
■ Verrucas and warts are removed by gradually abrading the infected tissue, and the same basic method is used for all preparations containing the above constituents:
– Before application, gently rub away the top layer of skin with a file, emery board or pumice stone.
– Apply the preparation directly to the top of the verruca or wart, taking care to confine it to that area.
– Cover verrucas with a plaster to encourage maceration and improve penetration of the medicament. (Some gel-based preparations do not require application of a plaster.)
– Remove the plaster after 24 hours (except for formaldehyde 0.75% gel, which must be applied twice daily) and file away the dead tissue on top of the verruca or wart.
– Repeat the process daily until all trace of the lesion has been removed; this may take up to 3 months and the verruca may regrow if all infected tissue has not been removed.

Silver nitrate
■ Silver nitrate is a caustic agent.
■ It is used as a stick or pencil (95% toughened with 5% potassium nitrate) to destroy warts, verrucas and other skin growths.
■ Unlike other treatments, silver nitrate pencil is used for only a short period – 3–6 daily applications are claimed to be sufficient.

Cryotherapy
■ Aerosols containing dimethyl ether and propane (DMEP) for freezing warts and verrucas are available over the counter. They are licensed not as medicines but as medical devices.
■ They are used daily for up to 10 days.

Self-assessment

Case study

A patient asks for your advice about a verruca that she has had for over a year. She has tried three preparations containing salicylic acid prescribed by her general practitioner and none has worked. She is now absolutely fed up and asks what she can do. What would your advice be?

Multiple choice questions

1–4. (Open-book, classification)

Questions 1–4 concern the following treatments for verrucas and warts:

a. Avoca
b. Glutarol
c. Occlusal
d. Posalfilin
e. Salactol

Which of the above:

1. is licensed for the treatment of verrucas only?
2. stains skin brown?
3. is contraindicated in pregnancy and breastfeeding?
4. must not be used for more than 6 days?

5. (Closed book, simple completion)
    Which one of the following statements relating to warts and verrucas is incorrect?
a. Warts and verrucas are caused by the herpes simplex virus type 1 (HSV-1).
b. Most verrucas and warts will clear up within two years without any treatment.
c. The highest incidence of warts and verrucas is in the 16–18 year age group.
d. Warts are usually painless.
e. Warts and verrucas are highly contagious.

Tips

In the registration examination, do not spend too much time on one question, especially in the open-book paper. Remember – no question scores more than one mark.

Gastrointestinal

Constipation	67
Diarrhoea	75
Haemorrhoids (piles)	83
Irritable-bowel syndrome (IBS)	89
Indigestion	93
Mouth ulcers (minor aphthous ulcers)	101

chapter 11
Constipation

Constipation is the infrequent or difficult evacuation of faeces. There is no exact definition, but it is a reduction in normal stool frequency accompanied by hardening of stools. Constipation that is not secondary to underlying disease or caused by factors such as side-effects of drugs or laxative abuse is known as simple or functional constipation and may be self-treated with advice from a pharmacist.

Causes

Constipation can be broadly divided into two types:
1. Simple (functional): constipation with no underlying pathology. There are various causes but it is often due to insufficient fluid or fibre in the diet, or reduced mobility. It can usually be corrected with dietary or lifestyle measures or short-term use of laxatives. Several drugs also cause constipation as a side-effect.
2. Secondary: constipation with an underlying pathological cause. It requires referral for medical investigation.

Epidemiology

- Constipation is common; it is thought to affect a quarter of the population at some time.
- Women are three times more likely to suffer than men.
- The condition is especially prevalent in the elderly, with up to 40% of people over 65 suffering.

Signs and symptoms

- Bowel frequency reduced below normal for the individual ('normal' can be from twice or three times daily to once or twice weekly).
- Straining in attempt to defecate, with possible abdominal pain and a feeling of incomplete emptying of the bowel.
- Stools are harder than normal.
- There may be abdominal bloating and discomfort.
- Stools may be specked with bright blood, due to bleeding from haemorrhoids caused by straining.
- Children with constipation may be irritable and lose their appetite.

Differential diagnosis

Causes of secondary constipation include:

- bowel obstruction
- carcinoma
- faecal impaction
- irritable-bowel syndrome
- hypothyroidism
- drug side-effects.

(See Symptoms and circumstances for referral below for further details of signs and symptoms of these conditions.)

Symptoms and circumstances for referral

- constipation for more than 7 days with no identifiable cause
- recurrent constipation
- colicky pain, nausea and vomiting, and abdominal distension (may indicate bowel obstruction)
- constipation accompanied by weight and appetite loss (may indicate carcinoma)
- blood in stools, which appear tarry and red or black (may indicate carcinoma)
- bright blood on stools or in lavatory pan. This usually indicates haemorrhoids, which is often not serious but should be diagnosed by a doctor
- alternating constipation and diarrhoea in elderly patients, which may indicate faecal impaction and overflow. In younger patients, alternating constipation and diarrhoea may indicate irritable-bowel syndrome
- constipation with associated weight gain, lethargy, coarse hair or dry skin (may indicate hypothyroidism)
- suspected adverse drug reaction. Constipation is a common side-effect of drugs with antimuscarinic actions, including:
- older antidepressant drugs, such as amitriptyline and imipramine
- antiparkinsonian drugs, such as orphenadrine, procyclidine and trihexphenidyl (benzhexol)
- antipsychotics, such as chlorpromazine and other phenothiazines.

Other drugs that can cause constipation include:
- opioid analgesics (morphine, codeine, dihydrocodeine)
- aluminium-containing antacids
- antihypertensives (such as verapamil)
- iron.

Treatment

Laxatives can be broadly classified into five groups depending on their mode of action:
1. bulk-forming
2. stimulant
3. osmotic
4. faecal softeners
5. faecal lubricants.

Bulk-forming laxatives

- Bulk-forming laxatives contain ispaghula husk (the seed coats of a species of plantain), sterculia (a gum from a tropical shrub) or methylcellulose (a semisynthetic hydrophilic colloid).
- These contain polysaccharides or cellulose derivatives that pass through the gastrointestinal tract undigested. They increase faecal volume through three mechanisms:
  1. adding directly to the volume of the intestinal contents
  2. softening the faeces
  3. adding to faecal mass by acting as substrates for the growth of colonic bacteria.
- They provide the closest approximation to the natural process of increasing faecal volume and are normally the first-line recommendation for functional constipation.
- They usually act within 24 hours, but 2–3 days of medication may be required for a full effect.
- They are not absorbed so have no systemic effects. They do not interact with other medicines and do not appear to interfere significantly with drug absorption.
- Adverse effects and disadvantages are relatively minor. They include:
- risk of oesophageal and intestinal obstruction if preparations are not taken with sufficient water
- abdominal distension and flatulence
- some bulk laxatives contain glucose, which needs considering in diabetes
- they may not be suitable for patients who must restrict their fluid intake severely.

Stimulant laxatives

- Stimulant laxatives are thought to act mainly by stimulating the intestinal mucosa to secrete water and electrolytes, through one or both of two mechanisms:
  1. inhibition of the sodium pump (the enzyme sodium/potassium adenosine triphosphatase), preventing sodium transport across the intestinal wall, leading to the accumulation of water and electrolytes in the gut lumen
  2. increased production of fluid in the intestine through action on cyclic adenosine monophosphate and prostaglandins, which promote active secretory processes in the intestinal mucosa.
- Stimulant laxatives may also cause direct damage to mucosal cells, thereby increasing their permeability and allowing fluid to leak out, increasing fluid volume in the intestine.
- The length of time for individual stimulant laxatives to take effect following oral administration varies according to their site of action, which may be in the small intestine, the large intestine, or both, but they normally work within 4–12 hours of administration. Doses are usually taken at bedtime to produce an effect the next morning. Suppositories produce much faster results, usually within an hour.

- The main adverse effects of stimulant laxatives are:
- griping and intestinal cramps
- following prolonged use, fluid and electrolyte imbalance and loss of colonic smooth-muscle tone resulting in a vicious circle in which larger and larger doses are needed to produce evacuation, until eventually the bowel ceases to respond at all and constipation becomes permanent. Stimulant laxatives should therefore be used for only short periods of a few days at most, to re-establish bowel habit.
- Stimulant laxatives are not contraindicated in pregnancy, but should be avoided in the first trimester. They are generally not recommended, and most are not licensed, for use in children under 5.
- Stimulant laxatives fall into two main groups: diphenylmethane derivatives and anthraquinones.

Diphenylmethane derivatives
- Compounds available are bisacodyl and sodium picosulfate.

Bisacodyl
Bisacodyl acts mainly via stimulation of the mucosal nerve plexus of the large intestine, so takes longer to act (6–10 hours after oral administration) than laxatives acting in the small intestine. It is minimally absorbed and appears to exert no systemic effects. It causes gastric irritation; there are therefore no oral liquid presentations and tablets are enteric-coated.

Sodium picosulfate
Sodium picosulfate becomes active following metabolism by colonic bacteria so it has a relatively slow onset of action, usually within 10–14 hours. It can be used in young children.

Anthraquinones
- Anthraquinones are naturally occurring glycosides used in the form of standardised plant extracts. They are thought to act through a combination of direct stimulation of the intramural nerve plexus and interference with absorption of water across the intestinal wall.
- Dantron and senna are the only anthraquinone laxatives in current use.
- Based on studies in rodents, dantron is believed to be potentially carcinogenic. It is a prescription-only medicine (POM) and is indicated for use only in terminally ill patients. It is available in combination with poloxamer '188' (an organic osmotic laxative) as co-danthramer, and with docusate (see below) in co-danthrusate.
- Senna is widely used.
- Senna is secreted in breast milk and large doses may cause increased gastric motility and diarrhoea in infants, so it should therefore be avoided by nursing mothers.
- Senna is excreted via the kidney and may colour the urine a yellowish-brown to red colour depending on its pH.

Osmotic laxatives

- Osmotic laxatives are either inorganic salts or organic compounds which are poorly absorbed and create a hypertonic state in the intestine. To equalise osmotic pressure, water is drawn from the intestinal wall into the lumen, raising the intraluminal pressure by increasing the volume of the contents, thus stimulating peristalsis and promoting evacuation.

Inorganic salts

- Inorganic salts used as osmotic laxatives are:
- magnesium sulphate
- magnesium hydroxide
- sodium sulphate.
- The effects of the inorganic salts are rapid: large doses produce a semifluid or watery evacuation within 3 hours and smaller doses act in 6–8 hours.
- Magnesium salts are also believed to act by stimulating the secretion of the hormone cholecystokinin, which promotes fluid secretion and motility in the intestine.
- Some absorption of inorganic laxative salt ions occurs but in normal, healthy individuals the amounts are too small to be toxic and the ions are rapidly excreted via the kidney.
- Accumulation of magnesium ions can occur in the presence of renal impairment, causing toxic effects in the central nervous system and altered neuromuscular function through hypermagnesaemia. As renal function tends to decline with age, elderly patients should be advised against regular use of magnesium-containing laxatives.
- Absorption of sodium salts can result in water retention and a rise in blood pressure, and chronic use should be avoided in patients with renal insufficiency, oedema, high blood pressure or congestive heart failure.
- The main side-effects of inorganic osmotic laxatives are nausea and vomiting.
- Large doses of inorganic laxatives can produce dehydration, so enough water should always accompany a dose to avoid a net loss of body water.

Organic osmotic laxatives

Lactulose

- Lactulose is a synthetic disaccharide.
- It is broken down by colonic bacteria, mainly to lactic acid, to produce a local osmotic effect and therefore takes much longer to act than inorganic osmotic laxatives.
- 72 hours of regular dosing may be required to produce an effect, which may be seen as a disadvantage by patients seeking rapid results.
- Lactulose has a sweet taste, which makes it more palatable for children, to whom it can be safely given, but many adults find the large dose volumes required (up to 30 ml) sickly and a deterrent to compliance.
- Serious adverse effects with lactulose are rare. Relatively minor side-effects, although they may be sufficient to discourage compliance, occur in about 20% of patients taking full doses and include flatulence, cramp and abdominal discomfort, particularly at the start of treatment.

- Lactulose is a disaccharide of galactose and fructose and includes some lactose, so cannot be used by patients with galactose or lactose intolerance and must be used with caution in diabetes.

Macrogols
- Macrogols (polyethylene glycols, PEGs), are condensation polymers of ethylene oxide and water.
- They are presented as powders that are dissolved in water and taken as a single daily dose.
- They appear to act more effectively and rapidly than lactulose, and have been suggested as the laxative of first choice for children.

Glycerol
- Glycerol is a highly hygroscopic trihydric alcohol that appears to attract water of hydration into the intestine. It is also believed to have a direct mild irritant effect and may have some lubricating and softening actions.
- It is inactive by mouth as it is readily absorbed and extensively metabolised in the liver.
- Glycerol is administered in the form of suppositories, which usually act within 15–30 minutes.
- It is a useful laxative for babies and young children.

Faecal softener
Docusate sodium
- Docusate sodium is an anionic surfactant that lowers the surface tension of the intestinal contents, allowing fluid and fat to penetrate, emulsify and soften faecal material for easier elimination. Evacuation is achieved without straining. It is also thought to be a stimulant similar to the anthraquinones. A laxative effect usually occurs within 1–3 days.
- Used alone docusate is a weak laxative, but it is considered useful for patients who must avoid straining, for example, following an operation or myocardial infarction.
- Docusate is non-absorbable and non-toxic but it is believed to facilitate the transport of other drugs across the intestine, and could thereby increase their action and adverse effects.

Faecal lubricant
Liquid paraffin
- Liquid paraffin is a purified mixture of liquid hydrocarbons obtained from petroleum.
- It is indigestible and absorbed only to a small extent. It penetrates and softens faeces, coating the surface with an oily film that facilitates its passage through the intestine.
- It has limited usefulness as an occasional laxative where straining must be avoided.

- It has several drawbacks that make it unsuitable for regular use:
- It can seep from the anus and cause irritation.
- It may interfere with the absorption of fat-soluble vitamins.
- It is slightly absorbed into the intestinal wall where it may set up foreign-body granulomatous reactions.
- It may enter the lung through aspiration and cause lipoid pneumonia.
- It should not be used in the presence of abdominal pain, nausea or vomiting and should never be used for children.

Additional advice

- To help prevent constipation:
- Eat a diet high in fibre, including wholegrains, fruits and vegetables.
- Cut down on food low in fibre, such as white bread, cakes and sugar.
- Drink plenty of fluids, the equivalent of at least 8–10 glasses of water a day. Hot drinks may stimulate bowel movements.
- Take regular exercise to improve digestion and bowel function and reduce stress, which can cause constipation.
- Establish a regular bowel habit. The best time to try for a bowel motion is usually the first hour after breakfast, when the gastrocolic reflex is activated. Be patient and sit for at least 10 minutes if necessary, regardless of whether you manage to pass a stool. Don't strain.

Self-assessment

Case study

A 75-year-old patient, who is generally healthy and whose only regular prescribed medication is for mild osteoarthritis, asks you for something for constipation. She says that she has never really had trouble with constipation before and wonders if it is just a consequence of getting old. On questioning she appears to be active, to eat a healthy diet including plenty of fresh fruit and vegetables and to have an adequate fluid intake. You check her patient medical record and discover that, because she complained to her general practitioner about having indigestion, she has recently been switched from diclofenac to co-dydramol for her arthritis. What would you do?

Multiple choice questions

1–3.(Open-book, classification)

Questions 1–3 concern the following laxatives:

a. co-danthramer
b. liquid paraffin
c. Movicol
d. Picolax
e. Senokot

Which of the above:
1. is not prescribable under the NHS?
2. is prescribable under the NHS but is not recommended?
3. cannot be bought without a prescription?

4. (Closed-book, assertion/reason)
   First statement: Magnesium sulphate is an osmotic laxative.
   Second statement: Magnesium sulphate is a poorly absorbed inorganic salt.

Tips

In the registration examination open-book paper, calculations section:
- Allow a maximum of 1 hour for the calculation questions.
- Do not get bogged down on an individual question. If you cannot work one out, move on; you may have time to return to it at the end of the exam.
- Do not get stressed or panic – remember you need only answer 14 questions correctly out of 20 to pass the calculations section.

chapter 12
Diarrhoea

Diarrhoea is defined as the passing of increased amounts of loose stools (more than 300 g in 24 hours in adults). There are several causes, but the condition is usually short-lived and symptoms can be treated with over-the-counter medication.

Causes

Acute diarrhoea (infective diarrhoea, gastroenteritis)
- Acute diarrhoea is caused by bacterial or viral infection, usually from contaminated food.
- Damage to cells in the intestinal mucosa causes inflammation and prevents absorption of water from the intestine into the blood stream, and the fluid is evacuated in watery stools.
- The condition is self-limiting and normally resolves within 72 hours.

Traveller's diarrhoea
- This is the term given to diarrhoea experienced by travellers or holidaymakers. Causes, and the severity of symptoms, vary with location.
- Attacks are normally short-lived, lasting up to 4–7 days, and begin early in a trip, although they can occur at any time.
- Some infections can cause persistent or recurrent diarrhoea and systemic complications.
- More serious microbial infections, such as typhoid and cholera, and parasitic infections, such as giardiasis and amoebic dysentery, may be contracted in tropical and subtropical areas.
- Up to 15% of patients with traveller's diarrhoea have dysentery (bloody diarrhoea).

Chronic diarrhoea
- Recurrent or persistent: there are several causes and chronic diarrhoea requires medical investigation.
- Causes include:
- irritable-bowel syndrome (IBS) – a common functional bowel disorder of unknown aetiology, of which diarrhoea is a common symptom (see Chapter 14)
- inflammatory bowel disease (for example, Crohn's disease, ulcerative colitis)
- malabsorption syndromes (such as coeliac disease)
- bowel tumour
- metabolic disease (diabetes, hyperthyroidism)
- side-effects of drugs
- laxative abuse.

Epidemiology

Acute diarrhoea

- The exact incidence is unknown, but it is very common and everybody is thought to have a bout at least once in their life.

Traveller's diarrhoea

- Between 30 and 80% of all travellers are estimated to suffer.
- In up to about 60% of cases no pathogenic cause is found. Of the rest, the causative organisms are:
- enterotoxigenic *Escherichia coli* – responsible for 40–75% of traveller's diarrhoea from an infectious cause; most common in Africa and Central America
- enterohaemorrhagic *E. coli* and *Shigella* species – up to 15%, most common in Africa and Central America
- *Salmonella* species – up to 10%
- *Campylobacter jejuni* – up to 10%, more common in travellers in Asia
- viruses (for example, rotavirus, Norwalk virus), protozoa and helminths – up to 10%
- *Giardia lamblia* (especially occurs in travellers in Eastern Europe)
- *Entamoeba histolytica* – up to 3%.

Signs and symptoms

Acute diarrhoea

- rapid onset
- watery stools, passed frequently
- resolves spontaneously within 72 hours
- there may be:
- abdominal cramps and flatulence
- nausea and vomiting
- weakness and malaise
- fever
- in babies and young children, diarrhoea may be associated with respiratory symptoms.

Traveller's diarrhoea

- early onset, usually within first 3 days of trip
- normally of short duration: mean 4 days, maximum 7 days
- bloody diarrhoea in about 15% of cases
- other symptoms as for acute diarrhoea.

Differential diagnosis

See Table 12.1.

Table 12.1 Diarrhoea: differential diagnosis

Feature	Significance	Possible indication
Frequency and nature of stools	Rapid onset. Watery stools, passed frequently	Acute diarrhoea Traveller's diarrhoea
	Blood and/or mucus in stool	Traveller's diarrhoea Inflammatory bowel disease
Occurrence	Isolated occurrences	Acute diarrhoea
	Recurrent	Traveller's diarrhoea Chronic diarrhoea
Duration	Resolves spontaneously within 72 hours	Acute diarrhoea
	Resolves within 7 days	Traveller's diarrhoea
	Continues beyond 7 days	Chronic diarrhoea
Onset	Begins within a few hours to a day or two after eating contaminated food	Acute diarrhoea
	Begins during or soon after return from visit to tropical or subtropical country	Traveller's diarrhoea
Timing of diarrhoea	Throughout the day	Acute diarrhoea Traveller's diarrhoea
	Early morning or during the night	Inflammatory bowel disease

Symptoms and circumstances for referral

- duration:
- more than 72 hours in older children and adults
- more than 48 hours in children under 3 years and elderly patients
- more than 24 hours in people with diabetes
- more than 24 hours in babies under 1 year
- babies under 3 months: refer immediately.
- diarrhoea associated with severe vomiting and fever
- history of change in bowel habit
- recurrent diarrhoea
- presence of blood or mucus in stools
- suspected adverse drug reaction
- alternating constipation and diarrhoea in elderly patients – may indicate faecal impaction
- signs of dehydration in babies: dry skin, sunken eyes and fontanelle, dry tongue, drowsiness, less urine than normal.

Treatment

Oral rehydration therapy

- The first line of treatment for acute diarrhoea is fluid and electrolyte replacement by oral rehydration therapy (ORT).

- Normal faeces contain 60–85% water, and the body loses between 70 and 200 ml of water per day through defecation. In diarrhoea, water loss of up to four times this volume per loose stool occurs, and sodium and potassium alkaline salts are excreted along with it, leading to a fall in plasma pH (acidosis). This can have serious metabolic consequences, particularly in the very young and the elderly. Fluid and electrolyte losses are increased if vomiting also occurs.
- Oral rehydration salts are not intended to relieve symptoms but are designed to replace water and electrolytes lost through diarrhoea and vomiting.
- They contain sodium and potassium to replace these essential ions and citrate and/or bicarbonate to correct acidosis.
- Glucose is also an important ingredient as it acts as a carrier for the transport of sodium ions, and hence water, across the mucosa of the small intestine, as well as providing the energy necessary for that process.
- ORT can be recommended for patients of any age, even when referral to a doctor is considered necessary.
- There are no contraindications unless the patient is vomiting frequently and unable to keep the solution down, in which case intravenous fluid and electrolyte replacement may be necessary.
- Fluid overload from excessive administration of ORT is highly unlikely, but possible if it is continued in babies and young children for more than 48 hours. Fluid overload is recognised by the eyelids becoming puffy, and is rapidly corrected by withholding ORT and other liquids.

Antimotility agents

- Non-prescription medicines are available containing the opioid drugs loperamide, morphine and diphenoxylate.
- One of the effects of opioid drugs is to cause constipation by increasing tone of both the small and large bowel and reducing intestinal motility. They also increase sphincter tone and decrease secretory activity along the gastrointestinal tract. Decreased motility enhances fluid and electrolyte reabsorption and decreases the volume of intestinal contents.

Loperamide

- Loperamide has a high affinity for, and exerts a direct action on, opiate receptors in the gut wall.
- It also has a high first-pass metabolism so little reaches the systemic circulation, and at the restricted dosage permitted for non-prescription use it is unlikely to cause any of the side-effects associated with opiates.
- It is not licensed for non-prescription use in children under 12 years.

Morphine

- Morphine acts promptly on the intestine (within 1 hour of administration), because of its direct action on intestinal smooth muscle and quick absorption from the gastrointestinal tract.
- Its action peaks within 2–3 hours and lasts about 4 hours.

- Morphine is not well absorbed orally and its availability may be reduced in combination products because of its adsorption on to other constituents.
- The morphine content of diarrhoea preparations may also be subtherapeutic.
- Morphine, particularly in Kaolin and Morphine Mixture, is subject to abuse and many pharmacists severely restrict its sale.

Diphenoxylate
- Diphenoxylate is a synthetic derivative of pethidine.
- It has little or no central action but acts selectively on gastrointestinal smooth muscle. It takes longer to act than loperamide.
- Diphenoxylate is combined with atropine as co-phenotrope. Atropine is included at a subtherapeutic dose to discourage abuse, on the premise that unpleasant antimuscarinic effects will be experienced if higher than recommended doses are taken.
- Co-phenotrope is not licensed for non-prescription use in children under 16 years.

Adsorbents
- The rationale behind the use of adsorbents is that they are capable of adsorbing microbial toxins and microorganisms onto their surfaces. Because these substances are not absorbed from the gastrointestinal tract, the toxins and microorganisms are thereby excreted in the stool.
- This lack of absorption also means that adsorbents are relatively harmless and safe to use, but there is little evidence that they are effective.
- Adsorption is a non-specific process and, as well as adsorbing toxins, bacteria and water, the drugs may interfere with the absorption of other drugs from the intestine. This should be borne in mind if recommending adsorbent antidiarrhoeals to patients taking other medicines.
- The adsorbents used in antidiarrhoeals are kaolin, attapulgite and bismuth salicylate.
- Bismuth subsalicylate is claimed to possess adsorbent properties, and some studies have shown it to be effective in treating diarrhoea. Large doses are required and salicylate absorption may occur. It should be avoided by individuals sensitive to aspirin.

Additional advice

For patients suffering from diarrhoea
- Drink plenty of clear fluids, such as water and diluted fruit squash.
- Avoid drinks high in sugar as these can prolong diarrhoea.
- Avoid milk and milky drinks, as a temporary lactose intolerance occurs due to damage done by infecting organisms to the cells lining the intestine, making diarrhoea worse.
- Many people with acute diarrhoea do not feel like eating, but those who do will probably benefit from eating light, easily digested food.

- Babies should continue to be fed as normal, whether by breast or bottle. Formula feeds should be diluted to quarter-strength, and built back up to normal over 3 days. During this period, babies should be fed more frequently than normal and feeds should be supplemented with ORT.

To avoid traveller's diarrhoea in areas of risk

- Always wash the hands thoroughly with soap and dry in the air or with a clean towel before using them to put anything in the mouth. Carry antiseptic wipes or hand-cleaning gel in case washing facilities are not available.
- Avoid the local drinking water, even for cleaning teeth; drink only bottled mineral water. Avoid ice cubes, dairy products, ice cream and home-distilled drinks.
- Eat only fresh foods that have been directly and sufficiently heat-treated.
- Avoid unpeeled fruit and vegetables and uncooked meat.
- Do not eat salads that have been washed in the local drinking water.
- Avoid shellfish and fish unless you are sure they are fresh and have not been living in water near to a sewage outlet.
- Avoid food from street stalls unless you can be sure this is fresh and cooked instantly.
- Try to eat only in establishments that are clean and hygienically run. Try to look inside the kitchen to ensure that there are no flies and no left-over food in pots, and that the staff have no visible sores or boils.
- Generally follow the dictum: cook it, boil it, peel it – or leave it.

Self-assessment

Case study

A customer asks for your advice about her 11-year-old son who has diarrhoea. In response to your questions she tells you that that the diarrhoea started yesterday after the boy returned from school, since when he has been to the toilet about six times. He has griping pains in his stomach but otherwise seems well. She says that he bought himself a takeaway kebab at lunchtime yesterday. Nobody else in the family has diarrhoea. What is your assessment of the situation and what would you advise?

Multiple choice questions

1–3. (Open-book, classification)

Questions 1–3 relate to side-effects of the following drugs.

a. aluminium-containing antacids
b. beta-blockers
c. carbamazepine
d. magnesium-containing antacids
e. non-steroidal anti-inflammatory drugs

Which of the above drugs is most likely to cause:
1. constipation?
2. diarrhoea?
3. indigestion?

4. (Closed-book, assertion/reason)
   First statement: Adsorbents such as kaolin are recommended for the treatment of acute diarrhoea.
   Second statement: Adsorbents such as kaolin may adsorb organisms and toxins causing diarrhoea.

Tips

In a multiple choice question exam, if a question stumps you, do not waste too much time on it. Leave it and go back to it at the end of the exam if there is time.

chapter 13
Haemorrhoids (piles)

Most cases of haemorrhoids can be managed by local symptomatic treatment, together with use of laxatives where necessary.

Causes

- The underlying cause of haemorrhoids is usually constipation.
- Anal continence requires the apposition of three mucosal pads, which are composed of three subepithelial vascular cushions that control defecation. Veins in these cushions fill with blood when sphincters inside them relax and empty when the sphincters contract. Any obstruction, such as constipation, may cause congestion and result in hypertrophy. Persistent straining, usually due to constipation, causes the cushions to prolapse and become enlarged. These prolapsed pads are haemorrhoids.

Epidemiology

- very common – up to 50% of people will experience haemorrhoids at least once in their lifetime
- rare in children and up to age 20: prevalence increases with age and is highest between the ages of 40 and 65
- common in pregnancy.

Signs and symptoms
- Haemorrhoids are often referred to as internal or external:
- Internal haemorrhoids cannot be felt outside the body, although there are other symptoms.
- External piles protrude below the anus; they may descend during defecation and shrink back again spontaneously, they may protrude and be able to be pushed back again with a finger, or they may stay descended.
- Symptoms of both types of haemorroids include:
- bleeding after defecation: blood may just stain the toilet paper or streak the faeces or, if copious, may splash around the lavatory pan
- faecal soiling of clothing
- mucus discharge
- pruritus ani (itching in the anal area)
- feeling that the bowel has not been emptied after defecation
- pain, usually with external haemorrhoids that have become thrombosed. This is often described as a dull ache that becomes very painful on defecation.

It can cause sufferers to ignore the urge to defecate, leading to a vicious circle of constipation and increasing pain. Normal sitting down can become uncomfortable or painful.

Differential diagnosis

- rectal prolapse – suspect if patient is female and elderly
- inflammatory bowel disease – can have various symptoms, some of which may be similar to haemorrhoids
- anal fissure: a crack in the wall of the anal mucosa, exposing the muscle layer beneath. It causes extremely painful defecation. Most common in both men and women between the ages of 20 and 30
- anal fistula: an abnormal channel between the bowel and another internal organ such as the bladder or vagina, causing infection and pain
- rectal carcinoma: most common in both men and women between the ages of 50 and 70, but can occur from the 20s onwards.

Symptoms and circumstances for referral

- symptoms present after more than 1 week of over-the-counter treatment
- recurrent episodes
- sharp or stabbing pain on defecation – this may indicate an anal fissure
- presence of blood. Bright blood does not normally have a sinister significance, but patients experiencing this for the first time should be referred
- blood mixed in the stools, giving them a tarry red or black appearance. This indicates bleeding within the gastrointestinal system and must be investigated
- large volumes of blood not associated with defecation; this may indicate carcinoma
- any accompanying systemic symptoms, e.g. nausea, vomiting, fever, loss of appetite.

Treatment
- Dietary advice on avoiding constipation is essential as this is the main cause of haemorrhoids.
- A wide range of products, in ointment, cream, suppository and spray formulations, is available without prescription for the symptomatic treatment of haemorrhoids.
- Most products contain a combination of ingredients. The main constituents are reviewed below.

Local anaesthetics
- Local anaesthetics used in haemorrhoidal preparations are benzocaine, cinchocaine and lidocaine.
- They reversibly block excitation of pain receptors and sensory nerve fibres in and around the area of application.

- They are weak basic amines with the same underlying chemical structure – an aromatic lipophilic group joined to a hydrophilic amino group by a linking ester or amide moiety.
- They reach their site of action by penetrating the lipophilic nerve structure in their lipid-soluble uncharged form, but exert their anaesthetic action in the ionised form.
- Local anaesthetics are included in haemorrhoidal preparations to relieve pain, burning and itching. Use should be restricted to the perianal region and lower anal canal; they should not be used in the rectum as there is little sensory tissue there and the anaesthetic can be readily absorbed through the rectal mucosa to cause potentially toxic systemic effects. Local anaesthetics are also absorbed through damaged skin.
- Skin sensitisation and systemic allergic reactions are possible with prolonged use, and use should be restricted to 5–7 days.

Astringents
- Astringents used are allantoin, bismuth oxide, bismuth subgallate, witch hazel (hamamelis) extract, Peru balsam and zinc oxide.
- Astringents coagulate protein in skin and mucous membrane cells to form a superficial protective layer. By reducing the secretion of mucus and intracellular contents from damaged cells they help relieve local irritation and inflammation.
- Some astringent substances, such as zinc oxide and bismuth salts, also provide a mechanical protective barrier on the surface of damaged skin.

Anti-inflammatory – hydrocortisone acetate
- Haemorrhoidal preparations containing hydrocortisone are available as P medicines.
- Use is subject to several licensing restrictions:
- They should not be used for patients under 18 years of age, or during pregnancy or breastfeeding.
- They should not be used for more than 7 days.
- The possibility of infection should be excluded because of the possibility of immunosuppression by the corticosteroid.
- They should not be recommended to new sufferers who have not consulted their doctor.
- Use should be reserved for the relief of pain associated with the inflammation of more severe haemorrhoids.

Other substances used in haemorrhoidal preparations
- Several other substances are used in proprietary haemorrhoidal preparations:
- mucopolysaccharide polysulphate – a fibrinolytic agent
- lauromacrogol 400 – a sclerosing agent
- shark liver oil – a skin protectant
- yeast cell extract – a wound-healing agent.

There is no evidence that any of these are of themselves effective in the treatment of haemorrhoids, although they and the bases in which they are formulated may have general astringent or soothing effects.

Administration and dosage forms

- The recommended treatment regimen for most preparations is twice daily, morning and evening, and after each bowel movement.
- Products containing hydrocortisone should not be used more than three or four times in 24 hours.
- The bases of all products are likely to contribute an additional emollient and soothing effect, and the lubricating effect of suppositories may ease straining at stool.
- Suppositories may slip into the rectum and melt there, bypassing the anal areas where the medication is needed and increasing the possibility of systemic absorption of local anaesthetics and hydrocortisone. This possibility is increased if the patient is lying down.
- Creams and ointments are generally considered to be preferable to suppositories for self-treatment of haemorrhoids.

Additional advice

- Give dietary advice on avoiding constipation, the main cause of haemorrhoids, which often results from a low-residue diet.
- Wash the perianal area frequently with warm water and a mild soap, or use toilet wipes, to reduce itching.
- Warm baths may reduce discomfort.

Self-assessment

Case study

A young woman patient seeks your advice about what she says is an embarrassing problem. You take her to the consultation area so that you can discuss the problem in privacy. She tells you that recently when she passes faeces she has noticed that there is often blood coming out as well. Very recently her anus has started to hurt; it is not very painful but it feels as if she is bruised on the inside. In response to your questions she tells you that she is generally fit and healthy, and she also tries to eat healthily, and tries to have lots of fibre. She wants to know what her condition could be and for you to advise her what could do about it. She says that she doesn't want to see her doctor about it as she does not want to be examined. What would you advise?

Multiple choice questions

1. (Open-book, assertion/reason)

   A patient brings in to you an empty tube of Anusol-HC ointment. She says that she got it on prescription from her doctor to treat haemorrhoids a few months ago. She went back today for another tube as she has haemorrhoids again and he suggested that she should buy it over the counter at a pharmacy because it would cost less than the NHS prescription charge.

   First statement: You do not need to send the patient back to her doctor to get a prescription for Anusol-HC ointment.

   Second statement: Anusol-HC ointment is a POM.

2. (Closed-book, simple completion)

   Which one of the following is not necessarily a factor for referral to a doctor of a patient who says she thinks she has piles?

   a. a sharp, stabbing pain on defecation
   b. blood mixed in the stools, giving them a tarry red or black appearance
   c. bright blood on the stools
   d. symptoms present after 1 week of over-the-counter treatment
   e. haemorrhoid symptoms with nausea and vomiting

Tips

For the Royal Pharmaceutical Society's registration examination open-book paper you need a thorough knowledge of the structure and layout of the British National Formulary, Medicines Ethics and Practice and Drug Tariff.

chapter 14

Irritable-bowel syndrome (IBS)

Causes

IBS is a group of bowel disorders, of which the characteristic features are abdominal pain or discomfort associated with irregularities in defecation, and for which no underlying pathology can be found.

Causes are unknown, but some possibilities have been suggested:
- abnormal bowel motility
- hypersensitivity of gastrointestinal tissues
- abnormal gastrointestinal immune function
- abnormal activity of the autonomic or central nervous system regulating the function of the gastrointestinal tract
- in some cases the condition may be psychosomatic.

Epidemiology

- Lifetime prevalence: 10–22%; IBS is slightly more common in women.
- Age at initial onset is between 30 and 50 years.
- Up to 70% of sufferers do not seek medical advice.

Signs and symptoms

- IBS symptoms fall generally into one of three types:
  1. alternating constipation and diarrhoea
  2. abdominal discomfort, bloating and constipation
  3. abdominal discomfort, faecal urgency and diarrhoea.
- There may be passage of mucus on defecation.
- Abdominal pain or discomfort may be relieved on defecation.

Differential diagnosis

Conditions with features similar to IBS include:
- inflammatory bowel disease
  (e.g. Crohn's disease, ulcerative colitis)
- malabsorption (e.g. coeliac disease)
- gastrointestinal infection (e.g. giardiasis)
- gastrointestinal carcinoma.

Symptoms and circumstances for referral

- age of onset over 45 years
- loss of appetite
- family history of carcinoma of the colon or inflammatory bowel disease
- fever
- nausea/vomiting
- symptoms worsening
- rectal bleeding
- diarrhoea unresponsive to treatment
- weight loss.

Treatment

Laxatives and antimotility drugs may be used to control diarrhoea and constipation.

Some drugs, mainly antispasmodics, are specifically licensed for treatment of IBS, and have been used for many years although there is little evidence of their effectiveness:

- Alverine citrate, a non-antimuscarinic selective antispasmodic that acts directly on smooth muscle, is indicated for the treatment of pain and smooth-muscle spasm in IBS.
- Hyoscine butylbromide, an antimuscarinic antispasmodic, is a hydrophilic quaternary ammonium compound that is poorly absorbed from the gut and claimed to act directly on it, and any drug absorbed does not readily cross the blood–brain barrier. Nevertheless, antimuscarinic side-effects have been very occasionally reported. Hyoscine butylbromide is contraindicated in patients with glaucoma, and caution is advised for men with prostate problems, the elderly and pregnant women.
- Mebeverine hydrochloride is a musculotropic antispasmodic claimed to act directly on the smooth muscle of the intestine without affecting normal gut motility.
- Peppermint oil: menthol, the principal constituent of peppermint oil, has been shown to have a relaxant action on smooth muscle. The oil acts directly on the colon and is formulated as enteric-coated capsules to prevent dispersal higher up the gastrointestinal canal. It may nevertheless exacerbate heartburn symptoms.
- Ispaghula husk, a bulk-forming laxative, is licensed for the treatment of IBS as well as for constipation and diarrhoea. It may aggravate bloating.

Manufacturers of some over-the-counter IBS products recommend that they should only be recommended following a medical diagnosis of the condition.

Additional advice

- Some sufferers find that eliminating certain foods and additives from the diet, including caffeine, alcohol, dairy products and artificial sweeteners, improves the condition.
- Stress-reducing measures and relaxation techniques may help some sufferers.

Self-assessment

Case study

A woman in her 40s who has been suffering IBS-type symptoms for several years asks you if you can recommend something as her diarrhoea seems to be getting worse and is making her feel drained and exhausted. When you ask if she has seen her general practitioner, she says not for several years, when he first told her she had IBS. What is your advice?

Multiple choice questions

1. (Closed-book, multiple completion)
   Which of the following clinical features is/are characteristic of irritable-bowel syndrome?
   a. bloated abdomen
   b. passage of mucus with stools
   c. passage of blood with stools

2. (Closed-book, multiple completion)
   Which of the following clinical features is/are characteristic of irritable-bowel syndrome?
   a. chronic diarrhoea
   b. chronic constipation
   c. chronic alternating diarrhoea and constipation

Tips

If you fail an attempt at the Royal Pharmaceutical Society of Great Britain registration exam, stay positive. Try to keep working in pharmacy for more experience and learning, and regard the next sitting as a new opportunity. Remember that the pass rate by the third attempt is over 99.5%.

chapter 15
Indigestion

Causes

- Indigestion (also known as non-ulcer dyspepsia or functional dyspepsia) is a term used to describe a range of symptoms in the upper gastrointestinal tract, with no serious underlying cause, generally associated with the ingestion of food.
- Two types of non-ulcer dyspepsia are commonly encountered:
  1. 'non-specific' dyspepsia, commonly known as indigestion
  2. gastro-oesophageal reflux, also known as reflux oesophagitis, gastric reflux or simply reflux, and commonly called heartburn.
- The common causative factor of both types is inflammation of the stomach and/or lower oesophagus caused by hydrochloric acid produced in the stomach.

Causes of gastro-oesophageal reflux

- Reflux of acidic stomach contents into the oesophagus is normally prevented by the lower oesophageal sphincter (LOS), which is situated at the junction of the oesophagus and stomach and acts as a non-return valve.
- Several factors can contribute to reducing the muscle tone of the LOS, allowing gastric contents back into the oesophagus, including:
- certain foods and drinks
- alcohol
- smoking
- some drugs
- obesity
- pregnancy
- anatomical abnormality.
- Unlike the stomach lining, the oesophageal mucosa has no protection against gastric acid and an irritant process ensues, giving rise to the characteristic symptoms of reflux oesophagitis – heartburn, a burning pain behind the sternum, and waterbrash, a sensation of acidic stomach contents regurgitating to the back of the throat.

Epidemiology

- Indigestion is very common: an estimated 40% of the UK population suffer at some time and 10% are thought to suffer on a weekly basis.
- There is little difference in incidence between men and women.

Signs and symptoms

See Table 15.1 for a summary of the clinical features of non-specific dyspepsia, gastro-oesophageal reflux and more serious conditions with symptoms that can be confused with indigestion.

Table 15.1 Clinical features of non-specific dyspepsia, gastro-oesophageal reflux and more serious conditions with symptoms that may be misinterpreted as non-specific dyspepsia

Feature	Significance	Possible indication
Age	• Age under 50	• Non-ulcer dyspepsia likely
	• Over 50 and dyspepsia for first time	• Consider possible pathological condition
Location	• From umbilicus up to sternum	• Non-ulcer dyspepsia
	• Behind sternum	• Gastro-oesophageal reflux
	• Specific point in abdominal area to which patient can point	• Pathology
Nature of pain	• Vague discomfort, aching	• Non-ulcer dyspepsia
	• Burning (heartburn)	• Gastro-oesophageal reflux
	• Gnawing, sharp, stabbing	• Pathology
Severity	• Mild	• Non-ulcer dyspepsia
	• Severe, debilitating	• Pathology
Radiation	• Localised to central abdominal region and epigastrium	• Non-ulcer dyspepsia
	• Radiates to jaw, neck, shoulder, arm	• Myocardial ischaemia
	• Starts centrally and radiates to right iliac fossa after some time	• Appendicitis
	• Radiates to back and shoulders	• Gallstones, peptic ulcer, pancreatitis
Associated symptoms	• Bloating, fullness, flatulence	• Non-ulcer dyspepsia
	• Regurgitation of stomach contents; burning sensation and acid taste in throat	• Gastro-oesophageal reflux
	• Persistent vomiting, blood in vomit, black tarry stools	• Peptic ulcer, gastric cancer
Aggravating or relieving factors	• Brought on by food	• Non-ulcer dyspepsia, gastric ulcer
	• Relieved by food	• Duodenal ulcer
Personal factors	• Stress, eating on the move, excessive alcohol	• Non-ulcer dyspepsia

Differential diagnosis (see Table 15.1)

- Gastric ulcer: becomes more common from middle age. Gnawing, constant, annoying pain in the mid-epigastrium, starting when the stomach is empty. Generally not relieved by antacids or food. Weight loss and gastrointestinal bleeding.
- Duodenal ulcer: incidence and pain as for gastric ulcer. Often wakes patient in middle of the night. Relieved by food.

- Gastric carcinoma: upper abdominal discomfort with nausea and vomiting, gastrointestinal bleeding, weight loss, dysphagia.
- Atypical angina: symptoms often difficult to distinguish from dyspepsia, but with general malaise. There may be radiation to jaw, neck and arms. May be brought on by exertion, cold or a heavy meal. Not relieved by antacids.
- Irritable-bowel syndrome (IBS): a common functional bowel disorder. Symptoms include abdominal bloating and pain in several abdominal areas. The cause is not known (see Chapter 14).
- Adverse drug reactions: many drugs can cause gastrointestinal disturbance as a side-effect. Those most commonly associated with indigestion include:
  - angiotensin-converting enzyme inhibitors
  - iron
  - macrolide antibiotics
  - metronidazole
  - non-steroidal anti-inflammatory drugs
  - oestrogens
  - theophylline.

Symptoms and circumstances for referral

- indigestion between meals or at night
- severe pain
- dyspepsia for first time over age 45
- dark tarry stools
- difficulty swallowing
- weight loss
- vomiting for more than 24 hours; blood in vomit
- pain brought on by exercise or effort
- pain radiating from central or epigastric areas
- suspected adverse drug reaction.

Treatment

Moderately raising stomach pH generally relieves indigestion symptoms. Treatment is therefore aimed at either neutralising gastric acid or suppressing its secretion.

Antacids

- Antacids have traditionally been the main form of treatment for indigestion.
- Several alkali metal salts are used. They are weak bases that dissociate to form alkaline salts, neutralising gastric acid.
- Antacids used in indigestion treatments have differing neutralising capacities, and the degree to which they are absorbed systemically also varies, influencing their duration of action. Soluble salts act quickly but are absorbed rapidly, so have a short duration of action, whereas salts of divalent and trivalent metal ions are insoluble and have a less rapid but more prolonged action. In addition some compounds form a protective layer

over the gastric mucosa. Antacid medicines are often combinations of two or more compounds, intended to optimise speed and length of action and minimise adverse effects.

▪ Antacid indigestion preparations often contain additional ingredients to control associated symptoms, such as wind, gastric reflux and colicky spasm.

▪ Compounds used as antacids are:

– sodium bicarbonate
– potassium bicarbonate
– calcium carbonate
– aluminium hydroxide
– magnesium salts
– bismuth salts
– magnesium–aluminium complexes.

Advantages and disadvantages of antacid compounds
See Table 15.2.

Table 15.2 Advantages and disadvantages of antacid compounds

Antacid compound	Advantages	Disadvantages and cautions
Sodium bicarbonate	• Effective • Fast-acting • Carbon dioxide generated during neutralisation of acid escapes through eructation (belching), helping relieve stomach distension that can contribute to discomfort of dyspepsia	• Highly soluble • Absorbed systemically • Prolonged use can lead to sodium overload and alkalosis • Excess sodium intake can lead to water retention, causing an increase in blood pressure and load on the heart • Products containing significant amounts of sodium bicarbonate best avoided by patients with hypertension, cardiovascular or renal disease, on a salt-restricted diet and in pregnancy
Potassium bicarbonate	• No possibility of sodium overload; used as an alternative to sodium bicarbonate in some preparations	• Hyperkalaemia possible with prolonged regular use in patients taking potassium-sparing diuretics or angiotensin-converting enzyme inhibitors
Calcium carbonate	• Greatest neutralising capacity of all antacids • Long-acting	• Safe in normal use, but problems may arise with excessive usage: calcium chloride formed during neutralisation of stomach acid is soluble and partially absorbed and can cause hypercalcaemia on prolonged use • Long-term use can cause milk alkali syndrome, with nausea, headache and possibly renal damage • Can cause acid rebound • Can cause constipation • Regular use of antacids containing calcium carbonate should be avoided by patients taking thiazide diuretics, as these reduce calcium excretion and hypercalcaemia may result

Aluminium hydroxide	• Forms an insoluble colloid with gastric acid; not absorbed to a significant extent and effective for much longer than a rapidly absorbed soluble salt • Lines the gastric mucosa and acts as a mechanical barrier against excess acid	• Used on its own, can bind to phosphate in the gastrointestinal tract, forming an insoluble complex; over a long period, may interfere with phosphate and bone metabolism • Tends to cause constipation, but often overcome by formulating with a magnesium salt, which has the opposite effect • Adsorptive capacity of aluminium hydroxide and its persistence in the gastrointestinal tract can retard the absorption of vitamins and some drugs, including tetracyclines
Magnesium salts (compounds used: trisilicate, hydroxide, oxide and carbonate)	• Tend to increase the tone of the gastro–oesophageal sphincter; useful in treating gastric reflux	• Absorbed to greater extent than aluminium salts • Excessive use, particularly in the presence of renal insufficiency, can lead to hypermagnesaemia, with serious cardiovascular and neurological consequences • Act as osmotic laxatives; overcome by co-formulating with aluminium hydroxide
Bismuth salicylate	• Coats the gastric mucosa, protecting it against acid attack	• Long-term use may lead to absorption and neurological damage • Absorbed and can cause same adverse effects as aspirin. Should be avoided by aspirin-sensitive individuals and in pregnancy • May be converted to bismuth sulphide in the gut, causing blackening of the faeces and tongue

Interactions involving antacids

- Antacids form insoluble metal ion chelates with tetracyclines, 4-quinolone antibacterials and penicillamine.
- They reduce absorption of tetracyclines and the antifungals, ketoconazole and itraconazole, as they are less readily soluble in an alkaline than in acid medium.
- They are also likely to reduce absorption of azithromycin, nitrofurantoin, rifampicin, phenytoin, chloroquine, phenothiazine antipsychotics and bisphosphonates.
- Antacids interact with enteric-coated tablets, capsules and granules, which are formulated to resist gastric acid and dissolve in the more alkaline medium of the duodenum, releasing the drug there. Enteric coatings may be disrupted prematurely in the presence of antacids, causing unwanted release of the drug in the stomach.
- Because antacids can interfere with the absorption of so many drugs, patients should be advised to leave an interval of at least 2 hours between taking a dose of an antacid and any other medicine.

■ Antacid preparations containing sodium bicarbonate should be avoided by patients on lithium therapy. Sodium ions are preferentially reabsorbed in the kidney, increasing lithium excretion and reducing plasma lithium concentrations.

Alginates
■ Alginates act as reflux suppressants.

Mode of action of alginates
■ Alginates precipitate out in the acidic medium of the stomach to form a sponge-like polymer matrix of alginic acid.
■ Carbon dioxide bubbles, generated by the reaction between stomach acid and the sodium or potassium bicarbonate included in alginate-containing preparations, become trapped in the matrix and make it buoyant so that it floats on top of the stomach contents like a raft (giving rise to the term 'rafting agents' for alginates).
■ When peristalsis occurs, the stomach contents are pushed up against the diaphragm and the alginate raft, which is claimed to form a physical barrier against the reflux of stomach contents into the oesophagus, is forced towards the gastro-oesophageal junction.
■ Aluminium and magnesium antacid salts are included in reflux-suppressant formulations because they help to neutralise stomach contents and any material that is refluxed through the LOS. Gastric alkalinisation is also thought to improve sphincter tone.

Antiflatulents, carminatives and antispasmodics
■ Additional constituents are included in some antacid preparations to:
– vent gas trapped in the stomach that contributes to discomfort (antiflatulents)
– act as mild counterirritants, producing a comforting warm sensation in the stomach (carminatives)
– relieve colicky spasm that is sometimes a feature of dyspepsia.
■ Simeticone is a silicone derivative; its surfactant activity helps to coalesce small gas bubbles into larger ones, which are then vented by eructation.
■ Peppermint and other volatile oils have surfactant and counterirritant properties. But they are also smooth-muscle relaxants and may aggravate gastric reflux by relaxing the LOS.
■ Dicycloverine and atropine are antimuscarinic drugs included in some indigestion medicines to relieve colic. They exert a relaxant effect on gastrointestinal smooth muscle and inhibit gastric secretion.

H_2-antagonists
■ H_2-antagonists available without prescription are famotidine and ranitidine.
■ H_2-receptor antagonists block the action of histamine by occupying receptor sites on the parietal cells. Histamine is the most important mediator of gastric acid secretion; it activates receptors on parietal cells, stimulating the activation of the enzyme hydrogen/potassium adenosine triphosphatase (H^+/K^+ ATPase), causing secretion of hydrogen ions into the stomach.

- H$_2$-antagonists exert their effect for much longer than antacids, as their action is not limited by the length of contact with stomach contents. Famotidine inhibits acid secretion and relieves indigestion for about 9 hours and ranitidine for about 6 hours, although they do not provide immediate relief as antacids do. However, an antacid and H$_2$-antagonist can be taken together for fast and long-lasting relief.
- H$_2$-antagonists can be taken in advance of consuming food or drink that is known to produce dyspepsia.
- H$_2$-antagonists are well tolerated and the incidence of side-effects is low.
- They should not be sold to patients taking non-steroidal anti-inflammatory drugs as they may mask symptoms of developing peptic ulcer.
- H$_2$-antagonists are not licensed for sale to pregnant or breastfeeding women.
- The activity of drugs that require an acid medium for absorption may be reduced by H$_2$-antagonists.

Omeprazole

- Omeprazole is a selective proton pump inhibitor; it directly inhibits the H$^+$/K$^+$ ATPase of the parietal cells of the stomach responsible for gastric acid secretion, and blocks the terminal secretion process of gastric acid. It has a more prolonged effect on acid suppression than H$_2$-antagonists and a short course can give up to several weeks' remission from recurrent attacks.
- Omeprazole is indicated for patients with chronic or intermittent dyspepsia, so long as there is no underlying pathology. Patients should be referred to a doctor if relief is not obtained after treatment for 2 weeks.

Domperidone

- Domperidone is a dopamine D$_2$-receptor antagonist with prokinetic and antiemetic properties. It acts primarily on dopamine receptors in the gastrointestinal tract to enhance gastric and oesophageal sphincter tone, gastric emptying and propulsion of intestinal contents.
- Domperidone is licensed for over-the-counter treatment of dysmotility symptoms of dyspepsia, including sensations of fullness, bloating, 'heavy stomach', trapped wind, belching and nausea.

Additional advice

- Advice to give to patients to help prevent indigestion:
- Eat regular meals and a balanced diet.
- Avoid smoking.
- Avoid excessive drinking.
- Avoid too much caffeine.
- Don't get overweight.
- Try to avoid stress.
- Eat small portions of food at regular intervals.
- Don't rush meals.
- Keep fried, fatty and spicy food to a minimum.

Self-assessment

Case study

An elderly patient asks if you can recommend something good for indigestion that she has had for the last couple of weeks. In response to your questions she says that she had been taking paracetamol for arthritis in her knees, but these had been becoming less effective lately and her doctor had prescribed some new tablets that were working wonderfully. You check her patient medical record and see that she has been prescribed diclofenac m/r 100 mg for the last 3 months. What will you do in this situation?

Multiple choice questions

1. (Closed-book, multiple completion)
   Which of the following drugs is/are H$_2$-receptor antagonists?
   a. nizatidine
   b. tolterodine
   c. zidovudine

2. (Open-book, simple completion)
   Preparation(s) containing which one of the following drugs *cannot* be sold without prescription for the treatment of indigestion symptoms:
   a. alginic acid
   b. bismuth salicylate
   c. domperidone
   d. hydrotalcite
   e. sucralfate

3. (Closed-book, multiple completion)
   If you are consulted by a patient asking for a medicine for indigestion, which of the following symptoms that he described would make you refer him to a doctor without investigating any further?
   1. He says he gets a feeling of acid coming from his stomach to the back of his throat.
   2. When asked where the pain is, he says 'right here' and points with one finger to an area on the right side of his upper abdomen.
   3. He says he has discomfort in his stomach that spreads right up to his jaw.

Tips

For the registration examination, make sure that you keep up to date throughout the year with important changes affecting practice, as the closed-book paper can include questions on recent changes in law and National Health Service guidelines.

chapter 16
Mouth ulcers
(minor aphthous ulcers)

Causes

The cause is unknown, but there may be a genetic predisposition, as about 40% of people with recurrent aphthous ulcers have a family history of oral ulceration.

Epidemiology

Mouth ulcers are relatively common, occurring in about 20% of the population, and in women more than men. The condition is uncommon in children.

Signs and symptoms

- Minor aphthous ulcers are small ulcers (5–8 mm in diameter), round and regular in shape, with a clearly defined margin, a floor of yellowish-grey slough and an inflamed outer margin.
- They occur on the sides of the cheeks, the tongue and the inside of the lips.
- They occur singly or in groups of up to five.
- Some sufferers experience a localised burning sensation for up to 48 hours before ulcers appear.
- Mouth ulcers heal spontaneously and without scarring within about 7 days.
- There is usually a history of recurrence.

Differential diagnosis

- Major aphthous ulcers: more than 1 cm diameter, in crops of 10 or more. They may coalesce into a single, very large ulcer. They heal spontaneously within 30 days.
- Herpetiform ulcers: pinpoint ulcers, in crops of up to 100. They usually occur at the rear of the mouth, and heal spontaneously within 30 days.
- Trauma: from biting the inside of the mouth or burning with hot food or drink.
- Oral thrush: creamy white plaques on the tongue and inside of cheeks. They can be scraped off to reveal raw red tissue beneath.
- Herpes simplex: a common cause of ulceration in children. It is difficult to distinguish from minor aphthous ulcers.
- Squamous cell carcinoma: initially painless, becoming painful over time. Mainly on side of tongue, mouth and lower lip.
- Chickenpox: spots often occur inside the mouth.

Symptoms and circumstances for referral

- children under 10 years
- duration more than 14 days
- painless ulcers
- fever or other signs of systemic illness
- ulcers more than 1 cm diameter
- crops of more than 5 ulcers.

Treatment

Treatments available for mouth ulcers are topical anti-inflammatories and preparations containing combinations of anaesthetic, analgesic, antimicrobial and astringent ingredients.

Topical anti-inflammatories
Corticosteroids

- Preparations available are pellets containing hydrocortisone sodium succinate 2.5 mg, and a paste containing triamcinolone acetonide 0.1% in carmellose gelatin paste.
- Corticosteroids are thought to exert their anti-inflammatory action through two mechanisms:
  1. stabilisation of lysosomal membranes, reducing the release of inflammatory lytic enzymes
  2. inhibition of phospholipase A, which reduces the release of arachidonic acid from phospholipids in cell membranes, inhibiting prostaglandin synthesis.

Method of use

- Hydrocortisone pellets: place one in the mouth in contact with the ulcer(s) and allow it to dissolve slowly four times daily for up to 5 days.
- Triamcinolone acetonide paste: apply to the ulcer with a finger, at bedtime and two or three times a day for a maximum of 5 days. Ensure that the area of application is dry so that the preparation can adhere to the mucosa.

Benzydamine

- Benzydamine hydrochloride is a non-steroidal anti-inflammatory and analgesic drug, available as an oral rinse and a spray containing 0.15% benzydamine hydrochloride.

Method of use

- 15 ml rinse or 4–8 puffs of spray every 1½–3 hours for up to 7 days. If stinging occurs, the solution can be diluted with water. The rinse is not suitable for children under 12 years.

Other preparations

- Several products are available in the form of gels, paints, pastilles and mouthwashes to reduce pain and discomfort (see Chapter 26 for an explanation of the rationale for their use).

- Some products are formulated as aqueous or aqueous–alcoholic liquids or gels. They tend to be diluted fairly rapidly and washed away from the site of application by saliva, requiring frequent reapplication. Pastilles or sore-throat lozenges containing a local anaesthetic, placed close up against lesions and allowed to dissolve slowly, may produce a more prolonged effect.
- An antiseptic mouthwash containing chlorhexidine gluconate 0.2% is available. There is some evidence that it reduces pain and the duration of episodes of aphthous ulceration. It is used undiluted twice daily.

Self-assessment

Case study

A man aged about 40 asks for your advice for a mouth ulcer. He says that he has had one for several weeks. He says that it has not really bothered him until recently, but it appears to be growing and has begun to get a bit sore. He says that a friend had recommended him to get triamcinolone paste, because it had worked well for him when he had a mouth ulcer. You ask to look at the ulcer, and the man shows you an irregular cratered lesion on the inner edge of his lip, about 1 cm diameter with some areas of blackening on the inner rim. Is triamcinolone paste a suitable treatment?

Multiple choice questions

1. (Closed-book, multiple completion)
   Which of the following factors described by a female patient aged about 30 would lead you to think that she is suffering from minor aphthous ulcers?
a. She has three whitish lesions, about 2–3 mm diameter, two on the inside of her lip and one on the tip of her tongue.
b. They are very painful, especially if she drinks anything hot.
c. She has had them before.

2. (Open-book, simple completion)
   Which one of the following would require a prescription in order to supply it to a patient for the treatment of mouth ulcers?
a. 1 × 10 g Adcortyl in Orabase
b. 1 × 15 g Choline Salicylate Dental Gel BP
c. 1 × 20 Corlan pellets
d. 1 × 10 ml Pyralvex oral paint
e. 1 × 16 Strefen lozenges

Tips

In the Royal Pharmaceutical Society registration examination, attempt all questions. There is no penalty for an incorrect answer, so even if you do not know the answer to a question you have nothing to lose by making a guess.

Infestations

Head lice	107
Scabies	113
Threadworm	117

chapter 17

Head lice

Causes

- Head lice (*Pediculus humanus capitis*) are small wingless insects that live on and feed on blood from the human scalp.
- Adult lice are transferred by close head-to-head contact for at least 1 minute or by using infested clothing, combs and pillows. Head lice may live for up to 2 days without a blood feed, and may survive for that length of time away from a host.
- Eggs are laid by fertilised adult females and firmly glued at the base of hair shafts. Nymphs emerge after 7–10 days and must feed within 24 hours to survive. The nymphal stage lasts 7–13 days. Fertilised females produce 250–300 eggs over the next 3–4 weeks before dying.

Epidemiology

- Head lice are endemic in the UK, with over 50% of schoolchildren aged 7–8 being infected at least once.
- Infection is most common in children aged 4–11 and more common in girls than boys, but adults can also be infected.
- Prevalence and resistance to insecticides are believed to be increasing.

Signs and symptoms

- Live and dead lice (about 3 mm long and greyish-white or brown in colour) and yellowish cast exoskeleton shells can be seen by combing the hair with a fine-tooth comb over a sheet of white paper, after shampooing and towelling dry. Lice faecal material (black specks) may be found on pillows and collars.
- Itching, an allergic response to lice saliva injected into the scalp to liquefy blood, may occur after several weeks of infestation.
- Nits are creamy-coloured empty egg cases that remain firmly attached to hair shafts as they grow outwards. Their presence is a sign of previous, but not necessarily current, infection.

Differential diagnosis

Dandruff and seborrhoeic dermatitis, which cause scaling and irritation of the scalp, may be confused with head lice infestation, but identification of lice material is diagnostic.

Circumstances for referral

When correct application of two complete cycles of different insecticides or other treatments has failed to eradicate infection, carbaryl preparations, which are prescription-only medicines (POMs), can be prescribed as fallback treatment.

Treatment

- Preparations of three insecticidal compounds are available without prescription to treat head lice infestation.
- A non-insecticidal treatment containing dimeticone is also available.
- Wet combing is a mechanical method of removing head lice without the use of chemicals.
- A head lice repellent, containing piperonal, is also available.

Insecticides

The insecticides (pediculicides) available without prescription for the treatment of head lice are:
- malathion
- permethrin
- phenothrin.

Malathion

- Malathion is an organophosphorus compound.
- It is a potent cholinesterase inhibitor that prevents the breakdown of acetylcholine and interferes with neuromuscular transmission in the head louse, paralysing it and preventing it from feeding. It is oil-soluble and absorbed by a process of passive diffusion through the lipid coat of both insect and egg; achieving a lethal dose depends on the concentration of the product and the length of contact.
- Malathion is poorly absorbed through human skin, and is much more efficiently detoxified by human metabolic processes than by those of insects. It is therefore safe for occasional or intermittent use at low concentrations as a pediculicide.
- There are no contraindications to the use of malathion apart from known sensitivity.

Permethrin and phenothrin

- Permethrin and phenothrin are synthetic pyrethroids with low mammalian toxicity.
- They are rapidly absorbed across the insect cuticle and exert their action on the sodium channels of louse nerve axons, causing initial excitement and then paralysis.

Dimeticone

- Dimeticone lotion has no conventional insecticide activity. It contains 4% long-chain linear silicone (dimeticone) in a volatile silicone base (cyclomethicone).

- It appears to act against head lice by coating the insects and thus disrupting their ability to breathe and to absorb and excrete water.

Wet combing ('bug busting')
- Wet combing is an alternative method for tackling the problem of head lice and resistance without the use of insecticides.
- The technique involves combing the hair while it is damp, with a fine-tooth comb for about 30 minutes after shampooing and using conditioner. If evidence of lice is found, the process should be repeated twice weekly for 2 weeks to remove lice emerging from eggs before they can spread and reproduce.

Piperonal
- Piperonal has no insecticidal activity, but acts as a head lice repellent. Its mechanism of action is unknown, but it is thought to provoke a negative response from the lice antennae receptors, causing them to avoid movement into treated areas.
- The main use is to prevent inadvertent reinfestation after treatment with insecticides, before all cases have been traced and the lice eradicated. It is not intended to be used as a routine prophylactic.

Formulations and methods of use
Head lice preparations are available as aqueous and alcoholic lotion, creme rinse and mousse and shampoo formulations.
- Malathion is available as aqueous and alcoholic lotions and a shampoo.
- Phenothrin is available as an alcoholic lotion, aqueous liquid and a mousse.
- Permethrin is available as a creme rinse.
- Dimeticone is available as an aqueous lotion.

Use of aqueous liquid preparations
- The solution is gently rubbed into the scalp, extending to the neck area and behind the ears, until all the hair and scalp is thoroughly moistened.
- The hair should be allowed to dry naturally, and the lotion left on for 12 hours, usually overnight. The hair is then shampooed in the normal way.
- While the hair is still wet after shampooing, it should be combed with a fine-tooth comb to remove dead and dying lice from the scalp and empty egg cases attached to the hair shafts.
- A second application after 7 days is recommended to kill any lice emerging from eggs that may have survived the initial treatment.
- The process is the same for phenothrin mousse, except that it is left on for only half-an-hour after drying before being shampooed off.

Use of alcoholic lotions
- Alcoholic lotions are applied in the same way as aqueous lotions. It is important that no heat is applied to dry the hair because the vehicle is flammable. The room should be well ventilated with no naked flames.

- Alcoholic lotions should not be used by asthmatics and young children as the alcohol may precipitate bronchospasm. Neither should they be used by patients with eczema as alcohol may cause inflammation and stinging.

Use of shampoo
- Malathion shampoo is much less effective than lotions and not recommended.
- It is more concentrated, but:
- – it is diluted between 15 and 30 times with water when applied
- – it has a much shorter time in contact with the hair and scalp
- – the insecticide may be inactivated by hot water.
- To use shampoo, the hair should be thoroughly wetted and sufficient shampoo applied to work up a rich lather and cover the entire scalp and neck area. The shampoo is left on for at least 5 minutes, rinsed off and the process repeated. The hair is then wet-combed.
- The procedure must be carried out three times at 3-day intervals.

Additional advice

- When head lice have been found, everyone who has been in close contact with the person in the previous weeks should be examined for lice by wet combing, and treated if necessary.
- Only those in whom current infection has been identified should be treated.
- Head lice preparations have no lasting prophylactic effect and their unnecessary use encourages resistance to the insecticides.
- Ensure that manufacturers' directions for use of preparations are followed closely. Incorrect use is often the cause of treatment failure.
- The mosaic model of treatment should be used to limit the development of resistance: as patients come forward for treatment they are each given a different pediculicide in rotation.
- Children with head lice do not need to stay away from school.

Self-assessment

Case study

A woman asks your medicines counter assistant for malathion shampoo for head lice. Your standard operating procedure for sales of P medicines instructs staff to refer to the pharmacist all requests for this product, which your assistant does. When you ask the woman why she wants it, she says that she has received a letter from her 6-year-old daughter's school that some children there have been found to have head lice. She is pretty sure that her daughter does not have them but wants to use the shampoo on all the family to make sure that they do not get them. How do you respond to her request?

Multiple choice questions

1. (Closed-book, simple completion)

    Which one of the following, used for treatment of head lice infestation, is a POM?

a. carbaryl lotion
b. dimeticone lotion
c. malathion lotion
d. permethrin lotion
e. phenothrin creme rinse

2–5. (Open-book, classification)

Questions 2–5 concern the following products licensed for the treatment of head lice:

a. Carylderm liquid
b. Hedrin lotion
c. Prioderm cream shampoo
d. Quellada M cream shampoo
e. Suleo-M lotion

Which of the above:

2. is not prescribable under the NHS?
3. is prescribable under the NHS but is not recommended for prescribing?
4. is a POM?
5. could also be used for the treatment of crab lice infestation?

Tips

There are no trick questions or traps in the registration examination, but you will need to use problem-solving skills to answer some questions.

Causes

- Scabies is a pruritic skin condition caused by an invasion of the mite *Sarcoptes scabiei*.
- The main symptoms result from immune reactions to burrowed mites and their products, such as faeces.
- Transmission is by skin-to-skin contact.

Epidemiology

- Scabies is more prevalent in children and young adults, but can occur in the elderly.
- It is more common in urban than in rural areas, more common in women than men and more common in winter than in summer.

Signs and symptoms

- Scabies is often misdiagnosed because of its similarity to other pruritic skin disorders.
- Sometimes greyish 'pencil-line' burrows can be seen, particularly on the finger webs, but they may be difficult to spot and obscured by excoriation due to scratching.
- The skin erupts in a red papular rash, on the finger webs first, then the wrists, armpits, genitalia, buttocks and abdomen. The face is not usually affected, except in children and the elderly. The rash is intensely itchy and scratching may cause excoriation and secondary infection.
- The itch can take up to 8 weeks to develop in patients who have not been infected previously, and they can be transferring the infestation to others while asymptomatic.

Differential diagnosis

- Bites from pet fleas or bedbugs may be confused with scabies, but these produce small red papules, often on the lower legs and ankles in the case of pet fleas.
- The rash may be confused with that of atopic eczema or allergic dermatitis.

Symptoms and circumstances for referral

- suspected infestation in babies and children
- secondary skin infection

- treatment failure
- unclear diagnosis.

Treatment

Scabicides
Scabicidal preparations available without prescription contain one of the following:

- Permethrin: a pyrethroid insecticide:
- The *British National Formulary* recommends the 5% cream as the first choice for the treatment of scabies. (The 1% cream rinse is licensed for head lice, and is not effective and should not be used for scabies.)
- Malathion: an organophosphorus insecticide:
- The same lotions are licensed for the treatment of scabies as for head lice, but the method of use is different
- Use of the alcohol-based lotion on skin damaged by scratching should be avoided, as it can cause stinging
- Benzyl benzoate: Benzyl Benzoate Application BP was once the first-choice treatment for scabies, but it can be unpleasant and has now been superseded by more effective products, because:
- at least two, and sometimes three, consecutive applications left on for 24 hours each may be necessary to eradicate mite infestations
- it has an unpleasant smell and can cause irritation, itching, burning, stinging and possibly skin rashes. It should not be used on skin excoriated through scratching.
- Crotamiton: an antipruritic with weak scabicidal activity:
- Up to five 24-hour applications at daily intervals are necessary for complete eradication of infections
- It is recommended for controlling residual itching after treatment with a more effective scabicide
- It appears to have a relatively long duration of antipruritic activity of 6–10 hours, requiring application only two or three times a day

Symptomatic treatments
Antipruritic topical preparations, including calamine and crotamiton lotions and systemic antihistamines, can be used to treat the itching.

Application of scabicidal preparations
- Correct application of scabicides is essential to ensure eradication of mite infestation. The method is similar for all preparations:
- The preparation should be applied with the hand, cottonwool, a small sponge or an 8 cm paintbrush to cool, dry, clean skin.
- The lotion should be applied to the entire body surface, from the soles of the feet to the hairline, including the head and neck, groin, axillae and skin folds, between fingers and toes, and under finger and toenails. Lotion should be reapplied to the hands if they are washed after application.
- Permethrin 5% cream needs to be left on the skin for only 8–12 hours before being washed off.

- Mites are usually killed within minutes of application of malathion preparations, but the aqueous lotion should be left on for 24 hours and the alcoholic lotion for 12 hours, to ensure complete eradication.
- Two applications, a week apart, are now recommended for both permethrin and malathion.
- Itching may persist for up to 2–3 weeks until the allergenic mite material is cleared from the skin, and should not be regarded as a sign of treatment failure. Patients should therefore be reassured and symptomatic relief offered if necessary.
- Treatment failure may have occurred if itching has not ceased after 3 weeks, or if new areas of itching are continuing to appear 7–10 days after treatment. In these situations, patients should be referred to their general practitioner.

Additional advice

- All those who have been in close contact with the infected person should be treated, as they may be infected although not yet displaying symptoms.
- Scabies mites cannot survive for long away from the human body, so bed linen should be laundered but disinfection is unnecessary.

Self-assessment

Case study

A woman asks for your advice about scabies. She says that she has just discovered that her niece has it and has been receiving treatment, but her children were with the affected girl last weekend and one even slept in her bed. She wants to know how likely it is that her children will catch it and if she should take them to the general practitioner for treatment as a preventive measure.

Multiple choice questions

1–3. (Open-book, classification)

Questions 1–3 concern the treatments for scabies and head lice listed below.
a. Carylderm liquid
b. Full Marks lotion
c. Lyclear dermal cream
d. Prioderm lotion
e. Psoriderm lotion

Which of the above preparations:
1. is licensed for the treatment of head lice but not scabies?
2. is licensed for the treatment of scabies but not head lice?
3. is licensed for the treatment of both scabies and head lice?

Tips

In preparation for any examination your revision should be methodical. Prepare a plan and a timetable and stick to them.

chapter 19
Threadworm

Causes

- The threadworm (*Enterobius vermicularis*) infests the human intestine. Reinfection and transfer to others are easily achieved by swallowing eggs.
- Fertilised female worms migrate down the colon at night and deposit their eggs on the skin just outside the anus. Eggs are picked up on the fingers while scratching the irritation caused by the secretions round the eggs. The eggs are then transferred to the mouth and reingested.
- Eggs can survive for up to a week outside the human host and can be picked up from almost anything, including lavatories, eating utensils, hard surfaces, towels, furniture and furnishings.

Epidemiology

- Infestation is common: up to 20% of all children may be infected at any one time and prevalence is up to 65% in institutionalised settings.

Signs and symptoms

- Night-time perianal itching, which may be intense and lead to insomnia and irritability.
- In girls, migration to the vagina can cause intense irritation, which may be confused with thrush.
- There may be anorexia and weight loss.
- Live worms (1–4 mm in length, white and pointed at both ends) may be seen wriggling on faeces in the toilet pan.

Differential diagnosis

- In adults, perianal itching may be due to irritation by deodorants, tight nylon underwear, haemorrhoids or perianal eczema.

Symptoms and circumstances for referral

- if infestation other than threadworm is suspected, particularly after return from travel abroad
- secondary bacterial infection from scratching
- in women, if there is increased frequency of urinary tract infections, vaginal bleeding during pregnancy, postmenopausal bleeding or abnormal vaginal discharge
- in males, if there is urethral irritation.

Treatment

Two drugs, both available without prescription – mebendazole and piperazine – are used to treat threadworm infections.

Mebendazole

- Mebendazole is the first-choice treatment for threadworm infection.
- It is a benzimidazole derivative, which disrupts parasite energy metabolism, irreversibly inhibiting glucose uptake and causing immobilisation and death of the parasite within 3 days. It also binds to tubulin, a protein required by the parasite for the uptake of nutrients.
- It is poorly absorbed from the human gastrointestinal tract, and the small proportion of a dose that is absorbed is almost entirely eliminated from the body following first-pass metabolism in the liver.
- Dosage for adults and children over 2 years is the same: a single dose of 100 mg. Treatment failures are rare, but reinfection is possible, in which case a second dose should be given after 2–3 weeks.
- Mebendazole is not recommended for children under 2 years.

Piperazine

- Piperazine acts by blocking the response of worm muscle to acetylcholine, causing flaccid paralysis. The paralysed worms are then expelled from the gut by peristalsis.
- Piperazine is readily absorbed, but is almost completely metabolised and excreted through the kidney within 24 hours.
- Piperazine phosphate comes as a powder in 4 g sachets, together with standardised senna, which acts as a laxative to facilitate the expulsion of the paralysed worms.
- It can be given to babies from age 3 months on medical advice only, and supplied without prescription to adults and children from age 1 year.
- Because the life cycle of the threadworm is about 30 days and some worms may be in the larval stage when the first dose is taken, the manufacturer recommends a second dose after 14 days to eliminate reinfection.
- Neurotoxic reactions resulting in convulsions have occasionally occurred in patients with neurological or renal abnormalities, and piperazine should not be used in people with severe renal or hepatic dysfunction or a history of epilepsy.

Additional advice

- All members of the household, even if asymptomatic, should be treated when a member has been diagnosed as infested.
- Employ scrupulous hygiene:
- The fingernails can harbour eggs; wash hands thoroughly and scrub under fingernails after using the toilet and keep fingernails short. Do not share towels.
- Wash all crockery, cutlery and cooking utensils carefully.
- Thoroughly clean all hard surfaces in the kitchen.

- Put underpants on children under pyjamas at night, to prevent them picking up eggs while scratching and thereby reinfecting themselves.
- Bathe or shower first thing in the morning, to wash away eggs laid overnight.

Self-assessment

Case study

A customer comes in to buy treatment for threadworm for the third time in 6 months. She says that her 6-year-old son keeps on getting infected even though she is taking scrupulous hygiene precautions. She has no idea how he keeps on catching it. What advice would you give?

Multiple choice question

1. (Closed-book, multiple completion)
   Which of the following statements regarding treatment of threadworm infection with mebendazole is correct?
a. The same standard dose of mebendazole can be given to everybody aged 2 years and over.
b. As reinfection is common, it is advisable to give a second dose of mebendazole after 2 weeks.
c. All members of a family or household should be treated, whether or not they show signs of infection.

Tips

Questions on some topics have been poorly answered in the registration examination. These are usually highlighted in the Royal Pharmaceutical Society pre-registration bulletins and it may be useful to give these issues extra attention when revising.

Musculoskeletal

Musculoskeletal conditions   123

chapter 20
Musculoskeletal conditions

Conditions for which non-prescription treatments are available include sprains, strains, sports injuries and mild rheumatic conditions. Low-back pain is often the result of these and a frequent reason for requests for advice at pharmacies for pain treatment.

Sports injuries
Causes

- Types and causes of injuries include:
- sprain: a sudden or violent twist or wrench of a joint causing the stretching or twisting of ligaments, and often rupture of blood vessels with haemorrhage to the tissues
- strain: injury to a muscle, often caused by overuse, resulting in swelling and pain
- fracture: a break in a bone or cartilage
- dislocation: displacement of one or more bones at a joint
- bruise (contusion): usually caused by blunt impact; capillaries are damaged, allowing blood to seep into surrounding tissue. Bruises are normally minor but painful, and easily recognised by their characteristic blue or purple colour in the days following the injury.
- Acute injuries occur suddenly while playing or exercising. Signs and symptoms include:
- sudden, severe pain
- swelling
- inability to place weight on a limb, hand or foot
- extreme tenderness in the area involved
- extreme weakness in a leg or arm
- a bone or joint visibly out of place.
- Chronic injuries occur as a result of prolonged or repeated sports or exercise activity. Signs and symptoms include:
- pain when playing or exercising
- dull ache at rest
- swelling.

Reasons for referral

- An injury should be referred for medical attention if:
- it causes severe pain, swelling or numbness
- a limb cannot bear weight

- a limb, hand, foot or digit is immobilised
- an old injury hurts or aches
- an old injury swells
- a joint feels abnormal or unstable.

Treatment

RICE

If an injury is minor, the RICE (rest, ice, compression and elevation) method to relieve pain, reduce swelling and speed healing can be used. Treatment should be started as soon as possible after the injury has occurred and continued for at least 48 hours, as follows:

- Rest: reduce regular activities. Take the weight off an injured foot, ankle or knee. Use of a crutch may help.
- Ice: put an ice bag or cold pack to the injured area for 20 minutes 4–8 times a day. A plastic bag filled with crushed ice and wrapped in a towel can be used. Remove the ice after 20 minutes to avoid cold injury.
- Compression: put even pressure on the injured area by binding, to help reduce swelling. A crêpe or stockinette bandage can be used.
- Elevation: put the injured area on a pillow, at a level above the heart, to reduce oedema.

Additional treatment

Oral and topical analgesics can be used to treat musculoskeletal pain.

Topical analgesics
Non-steroidal anti-inflammatory drugs (NSAIDs)

- Topical NSAID preparations containing benzydamine, diclofenac, felbinac, ibuprofen, ketoprofen, piroxicam and salicylic acid are available without prescription.
- The rationale for the use of topical NSAIDs is that they act directly at the affected site, avoiding the systemic adverse effects and side-effects of oral administration.
- Only a small proportion of an NSAID penetrates through the skin, but once absorbed it shows a strong affinity for tissues. Clinical evidence indicates that topical NSAIDs are effective over short periods for musculoskeletal conditions, are as effective as oral NSAIDs and have a very low incidence of adverse effects.
- Topical NSAIDs are licensed for the treatment of backache, rheumatic and muscular pain, sprains and strains, including sports injuries, and for pain relief in non-serious arthritic conditions.
- They are generally well tolerated, although side-effects associated with oral NSAIDs can occur, especially if large amounts are applied. Topical NSAIDs (except benzydamine) are contraindicated in patients who are sensitive to aspirin and other NSAIDs, and they are not recommended for use by pregnant or breastfeeding women or for children under 14 years of age. Clinically significant drug interactions are unlikely.
- Presentations of topical NSAIDs include creams, gels, mousses and sprays.

Rubefacients (counterirritants)

- Rubefacients are compounds that produce local vasodilation and create a sensation of warmth, exerting an analgesic effect by masking the perception of pain. Massaging enhances their effect and also helps to disperse local tissue pain mediators.
- Most proprietary rubefacient preparations are mixtures of several ingredients, including salicylates, nicotinates and counterirritant substances from natural sources, such as capsicum oleoresin, turpentine oil, camphor and menthol.
- Limited clinical evidence has shown that rubefacients may be effective for acute pain but moderately to poorly so for chronic pain.
- Products containing salicylates should be avoided by people who are sensitive to aspirin.

Back pain
Causes

- In many cases of low-back pain no cause can be determined. Contributory factors are general lack of fitness, and occupational and psychological factors. There are two main causes in cases where a mechanical cause can be identified:
  1. soft-tissue injury: strain of spinal muscles and ligaments (lumbago, fibromyalgia)
  2. trapping of a nerve root, usually the sciatic nerve, due to a slipped intervertebral disc (sciatica).

Epidemiology

- Pain in the lower back is extremely common: about 40% of adults claim to have suffered from it for more than 1 day in the last year.
- 60–80% of the population suffers from back pain at least once in their lifetime.
- It is most common in the 45–59-year age group.
- It occurs more or less equally in men and women.
- 90% of acute episodes of back pain resolve within 6 weeks.

Signs and symptoms

Soft-tissue injury

- Soft-tissue injury is often brought on by an event involving lifting or twisting.
- Pain may spread right across the back at the level of the top of the pelvic girdle, or may run vertically on one side of the spine.
- Pain may radiate to the buttock or thigh.
- Pain and restriction of movement may cause the patient to adopt a posture of leaning forward or to one side.
- The patient is otherwise well.

Nerve root pain

- Pain is felt in the lower back and often radiates down one leg, sometimes as far as the foot.

- Pain can be intense and burning.
- Pain is constant and made worse by movement.
- Patient limps and is unable to flex the hip very far, making sitting and climbing stairs uncomfortable; gait is stiff and awkward; patients may hold themselves rigid to avoid movement.

Symptoms and circumstances for referral

- if backache is not related to movement
- pain in the upper back not obviously due to muscle or ligament strain
- if associated with other symptoms of illness
- if associated with neurological symptoms such as numbness or tingling in legs or feet
- problems with bowel or bladder function
- severe pain at night
- cyclical low-back pain in women in the middle or second half of menstrual cycle
- no improvement with over-the-counter medication after 1 week.

Treatment

- analgesia with over-the-counter medicines (see Chapter 4)
- rest, particularly in sciatica, but not bedrest for simple back pain
- application of heat, e.g. hot-water bottle.

Additional advice

- Avoid stooping, bending, lifting and sitting on low chairs until the back is better.
- Stay as active as possible and continue normal daily activities.
- Increase physical activities over a few days or weeks.
- Backaches are rarely caused by a serious illness and usually go away in a few days.
- Stay at work or return to work as soon as possible.

Self-assessment

Case studies

1. A woman in her 30s asks you what she can do about the pain in her back. She says she is a cleaner and thinks the problem is the result of her work. She says the pain affects the upper part of her back on both sides and radiates round to the top of her ribs. What would you suggest?
2. A young man hobbles painfully up to the medicines counter and asks for advice about his ankle. He said that he hurt it in a tackle while playing football 2 weeks ago. He said that the team's coach had said he had sprained it and that it might take a few weeks to heal completely, and had advised him to use oral painkillers and a topical analgesic cream for the pain. However, it is still extremely painful and he cannot bear to put any weight on it. He wonders if there is anything stronger you could recommend.

Multiple choice question

1. (Closed-book, simple completion)

   Which one of the following constituents of topical analgesic preparations is a rubefacient?

a. benzydamine
b. felbinac
c. methyl salicylate
d. piroxicam
e. salicylic acid

Respiratory

Common cold and influenza   131
Cough   139
Hayfever   147
Nicotine replacement therapy (NRT)   155

chapter 21
Common cold and influenza

Two common upper respiratory tract conditions – the common cold and influenza – exhibit similar symptoms and are often confused by patients. Their features are compared in Table 21.1.

Table 21.1 Clinical features of the common cold and influenza

Common cold (infectious rhinitis)	Influenza
Causes	**Causes**
■ A viral infection of the nose, nasopharynx and upper respiratory tract. There are more than 100 causative viruses, of which rhinoviruses (responsible for 40% of infections) and coronaviruses (10% of infections) are the most common. Immunity to each is specific with little cross-protection; a vaccine is therefore impossible	■ An acute infection of the respiratory tract caused by three types of myxovirus. A vaccine is available, which is reformulated each year to keep up with antigenic shift in the viruses
■ Transmission is via nasopharyngeal droplets, released by sneezing and coughing, inhaled directly or passed on to fingers via surfaces where droplets land. Major sites of entry are the nasal mucosa and conjunctiva	■ Transmission is by droplet inhalation; it is highly contagious
Epidemiology	**Epidemiology**
■ It is extremely common: on average adults suffer 2–4 colds per year, and children up to 12 per year	■ Up to 15% of the population may develop influenza in any one year
■ Incidence is mainly in autumn and winter, but it can occur at any time of year	■ Influenza occurs in epidemics (400/100 000 population affected in a 4-week period) roughly every 3 years; and pandemics (worldwide epidemics) about every 10 years
	■ It normally occurs in the winter months
Symptoms	**Symptoms**
■ Onset is gradual, with initial discomfort in the eyes, nose and throat	■ Onset is rapid. Initial symptoms include shivering, headache, myalgia, vertigo and back pain. There is always fever
■ Symptoms are mild to moderate; they are uncomfortable and miserable, but the patient can carry on	■ Upper respiratory tract infection symptoms follow, including dry cough, nasal congestion and sore throat, although these are often less frequent and pronounced than in the common cold. There may also be anorexia, depression, nausea and vomiting
■ There is sneezing and nasal discharge (rhinorrhoea), usually followed by congestion	
■ There may be mild fever in children, but fever is uncommon in adults	

(continued)

Table 21.1 (cont.)

Symptoms Common cold (infectious rhinitis)	Symptoms Influenza
■ There may be sore throat and cough due to irritation of the pharynx and mucus dripping down from the nasopharynx into the bronchus (postnasal drip) ■ Recovery is usually within 4–10 days, although complications – laryngitis, sinusitis and otitis media – may follow and become complicated by secondary bacterial infection	■ Severe symptoms last up to 4–5 days. With no complications recovery is complete in 7–10 days, but lassitude, fatigue and depression can persist for several weeks ■ Secondary bacterial complications may lead to more serious respiratory conditions, such as pneumonia

Symptoms and circumstances for referral (common cold and influenza)

- Night cough in children. Fairly common in association with a cold, but in the absence of cold symptoms could indicate asthma
- Children with wheezing: may also indicate asthma
- Asthmatics: viral upper respiratory tract infections may trigger attacks
- Bronchitics: viral infection may become complicated with bacterial infection
- Cough persisting for more than 2 weeks, or becoming worse over a shorter period
- Dyspnoea: in elderly patients it may indicate cardiac failure
- Severe pain on coughing or inspiration may indicate pleurisy or pulmonary embolism
- Suspected adverse drug reactions, e.g. dry cough is a well-known side-effect of angiotensin-converting enzyme inhibitors
- Coloured sputum (yellow/green/brown), which indicates bacterial infection
- Blood-flecked sputum. Prolonged coughing may cause capillaries in the bronchial passages to rupture and spot the sputum, but there may be a more sinister cause, e.g. tuberculosis, carcinoma
- Noticeably raised temperature: this is a normal symptom in influenza, but refer if it persists for more than 48 hours
- Sore throat. Refer if:
- More than 1 week's duration, and/or persistent hoarseness, and/or dysphagia (pain or difficulty in swallowing) – may indicate carcinoma
- Dysphagia, and/or rash, and/or stiff neck – may indicate glandular fever or meningitis
- Suspected adverse drug reaction; sore throat is an early sign of drug-induced blood dyscrasias
- Earache. Nasal catarrh may cause a sensation of blocked ears and hearing loss. Pain usually means bacterial infection of middle ear (otitis media), which occurs frequently in children

Treatment

- Antibacterials are not effective or appropriate as both infections are viral. Patients with suspected bacterial secondary infection should be referred to a doctor.
- For influenza:
- Prophylaxis: vaccination is recommended for high-risk groups and all persons over 65 years. Oseltamivir and zanamivir may be used for postexposure prophylaxis and treatment under certain conditions (see National Institute for Clinical Excellence guidance in *British National Formulary*).
- Antivirals: zanamivir, oseltamivir and amantidine may reduce the severity and duration of symptoms, but are not a cure.
- The same non-prescription medicines are used to treat the symptoms of both the common cold and influenza.
- Proprietary over-the-counter preparations often contain a combination of ingredients intended to treat two or more symptoms.

Fever and malaise (see Chapter 4)

- Paracetamol, aspirin and ibuprofen can be used to reduce fever, if present, and ease headache and muscle pains in influenza and general discomfort with colds.
- Paracetamol, aspirin and ibuprofen are more or less equally effective, but there is often personal preference for one.
- Aspirin is restricted in its use by its pronounced side-effect profile, and may not be given to children under 16 years because of its association with Reye's syndrome, a rare but occasionally fatal encephalopathy in children.
- Paracetamol can be given to babies from 2 months of age and ibuprofen from 3 months.

Cough

See Chapter 22.

Nasal congestion and rhinorrhoea (runny nose)

Sedating antihistamines

- Sedating antihistamines are used to treat rhinorrhoea, exploiting the antimuscarinic side-effect of the drying-up of nasal secretions. They are usually co-formulated with sympathomimetics to counteract the congestion and the sedation that they tend to cause.

Systemic decongestants

- Systemic decongestants constrict the swollen mucosa and dilated blood vessels of the nasal passages, and improve air circulation and mucus drainage.
- Compounds used are sympathomimetic amines: pseudoephedrine, phenylephrine and ephedrine:
- They are central nervous stimulants and should not be taken near bedtime.
- They are contraindicated in patients with any kind of cardiovascular condition, diabetes or thyroid problems.
- They must be avoided by patients taking monoamine oxidase inhibitors or beta-blockers, as they can interact to cause potential large rises in blood pressure.

Local decongestants

- Sympathomimetic amines exert a rapid and potent vasoconstricting effect, confined to the area of application, when applied directly into the nose in the form of drops or spays.
- Compounds used are oxymetazoline, xylometazoline, ephedrine and phenylephrine.
- They can be used by patients for whom systemic decongestants are contraindicated, but should be avoided by patients taking monoamine oxidase inhibitors.
- If used for prolonged periods they can cause a rebound effect, with congestion often returning worse than before, and should therefore not be used for more than about 5–7 days.

Inhalants

- Preparations containing volatile substances for inhalation, either directly or via steam, produce a sensation of clearing the nasal passages and are used for the relief of cold symptoms. They have few, if any, contraindications.

Sore throat
Differential diagnosis

Sore throat is usually associated with the common cold but is also a symptom of more serious conditions that pharmacists should be able to identify and refer, including:

- Glandular fever (infectious mononucleosis): a viral infection, the features of which are sore throat, swollen lymph glands and fever. It is more common in adolescents. Patients normally recover within 6 weeks without treatment, but they may feel tired and depressed for several months afterwards.
- Tonsillitis: inflammation of the tonsils, usually caused by β-haemolytic streptococcus, with a purulent discharge, fever and malaise.
- Oral thrush (candidiasis): a yeast infection, causing sore throat and mouth, with white patches on the oral mucosa.
- Pharmacists must also be aware of drugs that can cause agranulocytosis through immunosuppression, of which sore throat is an early indicator. These include:
  - captopril
  - carbimazole
  - cytotoxics
  - neuroleptics, e.g. clozapine
  - penicillamine
  - sulfasalazine and sulphur-containing antibiotics (co-trimoxazole, sulfadiazine).

Treatment

- Sore throat treatments contain demulcents, antibacterials and local anaesthetics, and many products contain combinations of these. One sore throat lozenge contains flurbiprofen, a non-steroidal anti-inflammatory drug (NSAID).

Demulcents

- Sucking anything produces saliva, lubricating and soothing inflamed tissues and washing infecting organisms off them. Any lozenge or pastille, regardless of ingredients, will do this.
- Any non-medicated glycogelatin-based demulcent pastilles, such as glycerin, lemon and honey pastilles or boiled sweets, may be as effective as anything for soothing a sore throat. Because they contain no medicament they can be used as often as necessary to stop the throat feeling dry, thereby relieving discomfort.
- Some products contain ingredients with volatile constituents, e.g. eucalyptus oil and menthol, which produce a sensation of clearing blocked nasal and upper respiratory passages and can be useful in relieving other symptoms of colds.

- The main disadvantage of most demulcent throat lozenges and pastilles is their high sugar content.

Antibacterials

- The antibacterial compounds used in sore-throat lozenges are unlikely to be effective against the rhinoviruses that are largely responsible for the common cold. A sore throat complicated by a secondary bacterial infection, such as tonsillitis, would normally be treated with a systemic antibiotic.
- Gargles have the same drawback as lozenges insofar as most have no proven antiviral activity. In addition, contact time with infected tissue is extremely short. The main action of gargles is the mechanical removal of microbes from the pharynx, but levels of contamination build up again very quickly.

Local anaesthetics

- Benzocaine is the only local anaesthetic included in sore-throat lozenges; benzocaine and lidocaine are used in sore-throat sprays. A local anaesthetic may be helpful if swallowing is uncomfortable.
- Local anaesthetics can cause sensitisation in some individuals with prolonged use, so usage should be limited to 5 days.

Flurbiprofen

- Flurbiprofen is an NSAID available in a lozenge for the relief of sore throat. There is some evidence that it is effective and well tolerated.

Additional advice

- To reduce the likelihood of catching or passing on infection:
- If possible, stay away from people with colds or influenza.
- Avoid crowded places where the risk of infection is greater.
- Do not touch nose or eyes after being in physical contact with somebody who has a cold or influenza.
- Wash hands thoroughly, especially after blowing the nose.
- Throw away paper tissues after use to prevent the spread of infection.
- Keep rooms well aired.
- Treatment – common cold.
- There is usually no reason to see a doctor as a cold will clear up on its own within a week or two, and there is no prescription-only medicine that can cure a cold.
- Symptoms can be treated with over-the-counter medicines and warm drinks.
- There is no need to reduce daily activities, although sufferers should expect to become tired more easily.
- Sleeping with the head on a high pillow may help breathing at night.
- Avoid smoking, as it further irritates the throat and the lining of the nose.
- Treatment – influenza:
- Rest, preferably by staying in bed.
- Try to get plenty of sleep.
- Drink as much as possible, as large amounts of fluid are lost during a fever.

- Avoid smoking and drinking alcohol.
- Treat with over-the counter antipyretics and other medications as symptoms require.
- Consult a doctor if the symptoms have not gone after a week, or sooner if symptoms worsen.

Self-assessment

Case study

A woman asks you to recommend something for a very bad cold for her 74-year-old father. In response to your questions the woman tells you that he has had the symptoms for about 4 days, starting with a headache and pains in his back and legs and shivering, even though he said that he felt hot. She gave him paracetamol and after about 24 hours those symptoms subsided, but then he got a cough which is getting worse and keeping him awake at night, and she thinks he still has a slight temperature. When you ask about medication he is taking, she says she does not know exactly but says that he suffers from angina and high blood pressure. She says her father does not want to bother the doctor, so can you recommend something and let her know how long it should be before her father starts to feel better?

What would you recommend?

Multiple choice questions

1. (Open-book, assertion/reason)

   First statement: Amantadine is not prescribable under the NHS except as indicated in National Institute for Clinical Excellence guidance, when prescriptions must be endorsed Selected List Scheme (SLS).

   Second statement: Amantadine is not recommended for the prophylaxis or treatment of influenza.

2. (Closed-book, multiple completion)

   Which of the following would be factors for referral to a doctor of a patient whose representative asks for an over-the-counter treatment for an upper respiratory tract infection?

   a. a productive cough with clear sputum of 7 days' duration following a cold, in an adult

   b. a sore throat of 7 days' duration and no other symptoms, in an adult

   c. sneezing, coughing, sore throat and earache in a 5-year-old child

3 and 4. (Open-book, classification)

   Questions 3 and 4 concern the following drugs:

   a. adefovir dipivoxil

   b. amantadine hydrochloride

   c. oseltamivir

   d. ribavirin

Which of the above:

3. is a neuraminidase inhibitor?
4. is recommended for the treatment of influenza in at-risk children?

Tips

Do not be tempted to write everything you know about a topic in answer to an examination question unless the question explicitly requests it. You will only get marks for the specific information asked for, and you will be wasting valuable time by providing irrelevant information.

chapter 22
Cough

Acute cough is a common symptom associated with viral upper respiratory tract infections (URTIs) such as the common cold (see Chapter 21), and pharmacists are most frequently asked for advice and treatment for coughs from this cause. However, cough is a symptom of many conditions, most of which require referral to a doctor for further investigation. Pharmacists must be able to distinguish between a cough from a trivial condition and one from a potentially more serious cause and make appropriate referrals.

Causes

Cough is a reflex action to remove secretions or foreign material from the airways. In association with a URTI:

- in a productive or chesty cough, large amounts of cohesive mucus are produced in the upper respiratory tract as a defence against invading microbes
- in a dry cough, the inflammation and irritation in the pharynx caused by infecting organisms are perceived in the brain as foreign objects
- discharge from the nasal passages and sinuses flowing down behind the nose into the throat (postnasal drip) also causes reflex coughing.

Mechanism
Cough receptors in the epithelial layer of the pharynx and trachea are fired by the stimuli of excessive mucus or perceived foreign body and impulses are transmitted to the cough centre in the medulla oblongata of the brain. Impulses are sent back, via efferent neurons, to respiratory muscles of the diaphragm, chest wall and abdomen. These contract, producing a deep inspiration followed by a forced expiration of air, forcing open the glottis and producing the cough.

Epidemiology

- Cough occurs in 40–50% of symptomatic URTIs. On the lowest estimate of two URTIs per adult per year, this translates into nearly 50 million cases of cough per year.
- From sales figures it is estimated that about 25 million bottles of over-the-counter (OTC) cough medicines are bought per year.

Symptoms and signs of acute viral cough

- associated with other cold symptoms
- sudden onset

- usually more troublesome in the evening
- duration usually between 7 and 10 days, possibly up to 2 weeks
- any sputum (phlegm) is clear and colourless.

Differential diagnosis

Some of the more common and more serious causes of cough are outlined below. All require medical referral if suspected.

- Asthma: an allergic or autoimmune lung inflammatory condition, the principal symptoms of which are cough, chest tightness and wheeze. It affects about 5% of the population at some time in their life. Prevalence has increased in recent years, especially in children.
- Croup: a viral URTI occurring in infants and toddlers. The cough has a harsh, barking quality caused by laryngeal oedema and thick tenacious secretions that block the trachea and airways. Coughing attacks can be short-lived but are recurrent. In mild cases, sitting the child upright and steam inhalations are often effective. Serious cases may require emergency referral to the Accident & Emergency department.
- Whooping cough (pertussis): a bacterial infection affecting babies and children. Initial symptoms resemble a URTI, but paroxysmal coughing bouts develop which recur periodically for 6–8 weeks and sometimes for up to 4 months. The cough has a characteristic whooping sound. Attacks may cause the child to vomit and leave the child fighting for breath and exhausted afterwards, but between coughing spasms the child appears completely well. The condition can have serious consequences requiring hospital treatment and is sometimes fatal. Children are routinely vaccinated against the infection with diphtheria, pertussis, typhoid (DPT) vaccine, but it confers only 95% protection against pertussis and not all children are vaccinated.
- Chronic bronchitis is a long-term productive cough accompanied by episodes of shortness of breath. It is caused by chronic irritation of the airways by inhaled substances, most commonly tobacco smoke. Sufferers often have a history of acute chest infections that become more frequent and severe until there is a permanent cough.
- Heart failure: early symptoms of this condition of older people include a productive cough with frothy, pink-tinged sputum and breathlessness.
- Gastro-oesophageal reflux disease (GORD) (see Chapter 15). This condition is caused by reflux into the oesophagus of acidic stomach contents. The classic symptoms are heartburn and a sensation of regurgitation of acidic fluid up to the back of the throat. It may also be accompanied by a non-productive cough, especially when lying down.
- Carcinoma of the lung: most patients with this condition develop a cough which is productive and the sputum may be streaked with blood. Other common symptoms are weight loss, breathlessness and fatigue.
- Adverse drug reactions: drugs that can produce cough as a side-effect include angiotensin-converting enzyme inhibitors, non-steroidal anti-inflammatory drugs and beta-blockers.

Symptoms and circumstances for referral

- night cough in children: fairly common in association with a cold, but in the absence of cold symptoms could indicate asthma
- patients with asthma, as viral URTIs may trigger attacks
- patients with bronchitis, as viral infections may become complicated with bacterial infection
- cough persisting for more than 2 weeks, or becoming worse over a shorter period
- coloured sputum (yellow/green/brown), which indicates bacterial infection
- blood-flecked sputum: prolonged coughing may cause capillaries in the bronchial passages to rupture and spot the sputum, but there may be a more sinister cause, e.g. tuberculosis, carcinoma
- productive cough, with pink, frothy sputum and dyspnoea in elderly patients may indicate cardiac failure
- severe pain on coughing or inspiration: may indicate pleurisy or pulmonary embolism
- suspected adverse drug reactions
- cough with associated weight loss and/or fatigue.

Treatment

- All treatments for acute cough are available without prescription.
- There is no conclusive evidence either way on the efficacy of OTC cough preparations, but they are extremely popular. The placebo effect and reassurance derived from using them for self-limiting acute cough probably contribute significantly to their perceived effectiveness.
- Treatments are available for four types of cough:
  1. dry (irritating and non-productive)
  2. chesty with production of mucus
  3. wheezy, non-productive (no mucus is produced but there is a feeling of tightness or wheezing resulting from congestion of the bronchial airways)
  4. wheezy, productive (mucus produced, with bronchial congestion).
- The active ingredients of cough remedies fall into four main categories:
  1. suppressants (antitussives) to treat dry, irritating coughs
  2. expectorants for chesty, productive coughs
  3. decongestants for wheezy coughs
  4. demulcents to soothe any kind of cough.

Dry irritating coughs – suppressants
- Dry, non-productive cough serves no beneficial purpose and can justifiably be suppressed with antitussives.
- Two classes of compounds – opioids and antihistamines – are used as antitussives in cough preparations.

Opioids

- The compounds available are: codeine, pholcodine and dextromethorphan.
- Opium alkaloids act on the cough centre in the brain to depress the cough reflex. Both dextro- and laevo-isomers of opioid compounds possess antitussive activity, but only the laevo-isomers have liability for dependence.
- Dextromethorphan, a dextro-isomer developed as an orally active antitussive with little or no dependence liability, is the most widely used opioid constituent of OTC cough remedies.
- Evidence of the efficacy of codeine, pholcodine and dextromethorphan is conflicting, and most trials rate them as little or no better than placebo.
- Codeine and pholcodine have been traditionally rated as more potent than dextromethorphan, but have a greater side-effect profile.
- Codeine is partially demethylated in the body to morphine, which may contribute to its antitussive activity but also accounts for its liability to cause sedation, respiratory depression (although this is not normally a problem at OTC doses), constipation and addiction. Pholcodine has a generally better side-effect profile than codeine, and dextromethorphan is claimed to be virtually free from side-effects.
- At antitussive doses, opioids have no significant interactions with other drugs.

Antihistamines

- Compounds available are: brompheniramine, diphenhydramine, promethazine and triprolidine.
- All are sedative-type antihistamines, exerting a central and peripheral inhibitory action on neuronal pathways involved in the cough reflex.
- Side-effects include sedation, and anticholinergic effects such as dry mouth, urinary retention, constipation and blurring of vision. Both types of side-effect may be useful in cough preparations, aiding sleep if taken near to bedtime and drying up bronchial and nasal secretions.
- Because of side-effects, cough preparations containing antihistamines should not be recommended to patients with glaucoma or prostate problems and should be used with caution in older patients.
- Interactions: the sedative effects of antidepressants, anxiolytics and hypnotics are likely to be enhanced by antihistamines, as are the antimuscarinic actions and side-effects of drugs such as trihexyphenidyl, orphenadrine, tricyclic antidepressants and phenothiazines.

Chesty, productive coughs – expectorants

- Compounds available are: guaifenesin, ammonium chloride, ipecacuanha and squill.
- In productive cough, mucus produced in the bronchial passages as a result of infection is moved upwards towards the pharynx by ciliary action and is then expelled by coughing. As the cough is clearing mucus and helping to keep the airways open, it should not be suppressed.
- Expectorants are used to assist mucus removal. In large doses they are emetic, acting through vagal stimulation of the gastric mucosa to produce a

reflex response from the vomiting centre in the brain. The same mechanism stimulates the bronchial glands and cilia and it is postulated that this stimulation still occurs at subemetic doses.

- Expectorants have long been used in the treatment of cough, but there is little objective evidence of their effectiveness.
- Guaifenesin is the expectorant most frequently used in proprietary preparations, and is the only one recognised to have any activity.
- Many expectorant preparations contain what appear to be subtherapeutic levels of constituents.
- There is little risk of adverse effects from expectorants and they do not interact with other drugs.

Wheezy coughs – decongestants

- The sympathomimetics ephedrine and pseudoephedrine are used as decongestants and bronchodilators in cough remedies.
- Sympathomimetics mimic the action of noradrenaline (norepinephrine), the principal neurotransmitter between the nerve endings of the sympathetic nervous system and the adrenergic receptors of the innervated tissues. They stimulate both alpha-adrenoceptors, causing constriction of smooth muscle and blood vessels, and beta-adrenoceptors, producing bronchodilatation. They are therefore useful in coughs where the tissues of the upper respiratory tract are congested, as they shrink swollen mucosa and open up the airways.
- Ephedrine and pseudoephedrine have more or less equivalent action on the respiratory tract, but ephedrine has greater central nervous system and pressor activity and is used in few products.
- Adverse drug reactions: because of their pressor effects, and because they can also increase heart rate, sympathomimetic decongestants should be avoided by patients with any kind of cardiovascular condition or glaucoma. They also interfere with metabolism, including glucose metabolism, and should not be taken by patients with diabetes or thyroid problems. As they are central nervous system stimulants, doses should not be taken near to bedtime.
- Sympathomimetic decongestants interact with monoamine oxidase inhibitors (MAOIs), preventing the breakdown of noradrenaline and increasing the amount stored in adrenergic nerve terminals. Administration of a sympathomimetic with an MAOI increases the level of adrenergic transmitter substances, and can result in potentially lethal hypertensive crises. Sympathomimetic decongestants must therefore not be given to patients taking MAOIs.
- Oral decongestants should also be avoided by patients taking beta-blockers, as sympathomimetics stimulate both the alpha-adrenoceptors of the cardiovascular system to produce vasoconstriction and the beta-adrenoceptors to produce vasodilatation and stimulation of the heart. The overall effect is a slight increase in both blood pressure and heart rate. If the beta-receptors are blocked, unopposed alpha-adrenoceptor-mediated vasoconstriction can lead to a rise in blood pressure.

- (A methylxanthine, theophylline, is used in one proprietary OTC preparation marketed for the treatment of bronchial cough, breathlessness and wheezing. It is now little used and its side-effects and interactions make it unsuitable for recommendation.)

Treatment for any kind of cough – demulcents

- Demulcents coat the mucosa of the pharynx and provide short-lived relief of the irritation that provokes reflex coughing. They are mainly used for their placebo effect, although a possible true pharmacological effect has been proposed.
- Compounds used in demulcent cough remedies include: glycerol, liquid glucose, syrup, honey and treacle.
- Pastilles (e.g. glycerin, lemon and honey) provide a more prolonged soothing effect than liquids as they promote production of saliva, which has a demulcent effect, while the pastille is being sucked.
- Demulcents can be safely taken by anyone, the only drawback being the high sugar content of some preparations, which should be used with caution in patients with diabetes, and in children because of their cariogenic potential. Several sugar-free linctuses are available.

Combination products

- Some cough remedies contain just an antitussive (usually dextromethorphan) or an expectorant (usually guaifenesin), but the majority are mixtures containing up to six ingredients, plus vehicle and flavourings.
- Many products contain pharmacologically rational combinations, such as an antitussive with a decongestant/bronchodilator, which is sensible for a dry cough with wheeziness or congestion, or an expectorant with a decongestant, suitable for a productive cough with congestion.
- There are, however, a few irrational formulations that combine an expectorant with an antihistamine and which have mutually antagonistic effects on clearance of mucus, or that combine an antitussive to suppress coughing with an expectorant to promote it.
- Some products contain mixtures of several ingredients of doubtful efficacy in subtherapeutic amounts.

Self-assessment

Case study

A woman asks you for advice about her 6-year old son's cough. He had a chest infection a month ago, for which he was given antibiotics. It cleared up but he has had a cough again for about the last week. He has had this type of cough a couple of times before, but it has gone away of its own accord. The woman asks if her son could have developed an allergy to something and if that is what is causing the cough.

Multiple choice questions

1. (Open-book, simple completion)

    A nurse prescriber asks you to advise her on what she should prescribe for a non-productive cough for a 4-year-old child with a URTI. Of the following, which one would you suggest?

a. Benylin paediatric
b. Buttercup syrup
c. Galenphol paediatric linctus
d. Meltus junior expectorant
e. Simple paediatric linctus

2–4. (Closed-book, classification)

   Questions 2–4 relate to the following conditions:

a. asthma
b. congestive heart failure
c. GORD
d. lung carcinoma
e. URTI

   Which of the conditions above are suggested by the following scenarios?

2. A middle-aged man asks for something for persistent heartburn. He also wants something for a dry cough.
3. An elderly lady asks for something for her cough. On questioning she tells you that she has had it for a few weeks, is bringing up frothy sputum and feels a bit out of breath.
4. A young woman asks for something for her boyfriend, who is at home. He has had a sore throat, followed by sneezing and a runny nose. He now has a cough, and he says he feels like he has something on his chest but can't bring it up.

Tips

In assertion/reason questions in the pre-registration examination, discriminate carefully between keys A and B. A is the correct answer if the two statements are correct and can be linked with the word 'because'.

chapter 23
Hayfever

Seasonal allergic rhinitis and/or conjunctivitis, more commonly known as hayfever, are allergic hypersensitivity reactions in the nasal mucosa and the conjunctiva of the eye associated with the presence of pollens in the atmosphere in the summer months.

Causes

- Hayfever is caused by exposure to pollen or other allergens that only occur at certain times of year. The most common causes are:
- tree pollens in spring
- grass pollen in summer
- mugwort and chrysanthemum pollen and fungal spores in autumn.
- Symptoms are the result of a type I allergic reaction in which initial exposure of a sensitive individual to an antigen results in the production of antigen-specific immunoglobulin E (IgE). IgE attaches to mast cells and basophils, which become sensitive to further antigenic material. On further exposure the antigen binds to IgE, causing degranulation of the mast cells and release of chemical mediators, including histamine, leukotrienes and prostaglandins, which produce an inflammatory response. Prolonged exposure to the allergen may result in a sustained response, causing nasal congestion.

Epidemiology

- Hayfever is estimated to affect 10–15% of the UK population, and the incidence appears to be rising.
- Up to 10% of children and 20–30% of adolescents are thought to suffer. Incidence peaks in the early teens and then diminishes. About two-thirds of adult sufferers are under 30 years old.
- Heredity may play a role, and children whose parents suffer from hayfever have a high chance of suffering themselves.

Signs and symptoms

Nasal symptoms
The development of nasal symptoms over time is described in terms of early and late phases.

Early-phase nasal symptoms

- Rhinorrhoea (nasal discharge): discharge is clear and watery, and frequent blowing and wiping can make the nose sore, sometimes leading to infections.
- Sneezing: begins within 60 seconds of inhalation of allergen and can result in long bouts of repeated sneezing, which is disruptive and distressing.
- Nasal pruritus (itching): may be continuous or intermittent, and is extremely unpleasant and irritating.
- Some sufferers also experience an itching sensation in the roof of the mouth.

Late-phase nasal symptoms

- Nasal congestion, usually developing after some days of exposure to allergen, when the blood vessels in the nose become dilated. Congestion may be uni- or bilateral, and may shift from one nostril to the other every few hours. Mouth-breathing may result, which can lead to a dry mouth and bad breath, disrupted sleep and anosmia (loss of sense of smell).
- Nasal congestion may cause frontal or sinus headaches and give rise to secondary infections such as sinusitis.
- The eustachian tubes may become blocked with mucus and infected, and otitis media may result.
- In some cases a dark or bluish swelling, like a black eye, develops around the eyes, caused by impaired nasal venous outflow.

Eye symptoms: allergic conjunctivitis

- clear, watery ophthalmic discharge
- redness caused by dilation of the conjunctival blood vessels
- ophthalmic itching, sometimes so severe that the sufferer resorts to scratching the eyelids to relieve it
- photophobia
- skin folds or pleats develop parallel to the lower lid margin, extending from under the eye to the top of the cheekbone.

Differential diagnosis

Allergic rhinitis and the common cold have several features in common. They may be confused with each other but can be distinguished by the differences shown in Table 23.1.

Symptoms and circumstances for referral

- wheezing or shortness of breath, which could indicate asthma
- earache or facial pain, as these may indicate sinusitis or otitis media requiring antibiotics
- purulent, rather than clear, discharge from the eyes, indicating the possibility of infection
- blood in nasal discharge
- no improvement after 1 week of treatment with over-the-counter medication.

Table 23.1 Differential diagnosis of hayfever (allergic rhinitis) and the common cold

Allergic rhinitis	Common cold
Nasal discharge usually remains clear, and if it does become infected takes much longer to do so	The initially clear nasal discharge usually thickens and becomes purulent within a few days
Sneezing usually frequent and paroxysmal	Sneezing usually less frequent
Nasal itching common	Normally no nasal itching
Eye symptoms common	Normally no eye symptoms
Symptoms continue for as long as the sufferer is affected by the allergen, often several weeks	Symptoms last for about 4–7 days
Sudden onset of symptoms	Gradual onset of symptoms
Symptoms occur at the same time each year, when the causative allergen is in the air	Can occur any time, but more usually in the winter
Affects only isolated individuals	Highly contagious; other family members or acquaintances may be suffering at the same time and the infection will be quite common in the community

Treatment

Systemic treatment

- Histamine is the main chemical mediator responsible for the inflammatory response of hayfever and other allergic reactions. All oral formulations for treatment of hayfever are antihistamines and act through competitive antagonism of histamine at the H_1-receptor.
- Antihistamines are generally effective in controlling symptoms of hayfever, including sneezing, nasal itching, rhinorrhoea and, to a lesser extent, allergic conjunctivitis, but they have little or no effect on nasal congestion.
- The maximum effect of antihistamines is not achieved until several hours after peak serum levels have been reached and they cannot reverse the consequences of H_1-receptor activation, so are only effective if they are able to block histamine release before it occurs. For maximum effectiveness, therefore, antihistamines should be taken when symptoms are expected, rather than after they have started.
- Oral antihistamines fall into two groups: sedating and non-sedating.

Sedating antihistamines

- Sedating antihistamines (also known as first-generation antihistamines):
- are lipophilic and readily cross the blood–brain barrier
- as well as binding to H_1-receptors, bind to and block muscarinic receptors and, in some cases, alpha-adrenergic and serotonergic receptors in the brain, and, as a result
- can cause several generally undesirable side-effects, including sedation, dry mouth, blurred vision, urinary retention, constipation and gastrointestinal disturbances.
- Sedating antihitamines available without prescription are:
- chlorphenamine
- clemastine
- diphenhydramine
- promethazine.

- There is no evidence of difference in effectiveness between older antihistamines, although individual response to specific drugs varies widely. Choice is often based on personal preference and factors such as the degree of sedation caused and duration of action, which do differ between compounds.

Non-sedating antihistamines
- In comparison with sedating antihistamines, non-sedating antihistamines (also known as second-generation):
- are less lipophilic and do not reach the brain to a significant extent
- are much less likely to cause centrally mediated adverse side-effects. (However, a few individuals exhibit drowsiness and other central nervous system side-effects in response to non-sedating antihistamines and even to placebo, and impairment of function, if it occurs, is not always accompanied by subjective feelings of drowsiness. Patients should therefore be warned that these antihistamines may affect driving and other skilled tasks and that excess alcohol should be avoided.)
- Compounds available are:
- acrivastine
- cetirizine
- loratadine.
  All are of equal efficacy.
- Acrivastine has a rapid onset of action and a short half-life, necessitating more frequent dosing than cetirizine or loratadine, but it may be useful to give rapid relief.
- Peak plasma levels of cetirizine and loratadine are reached in about an hour; they have long elimination half-lives and are long-acting, requiring only once-daily dosage.
- The incidence of sedation is extremely low for all three drugs, but loratadine is less likely to be sedating than acrivastine or cetirizine.

Combination products
- Some oral products combine antihistamines with sympathomimetic decongestants and are marketed for nasal congestion associated with hayfever and the common cold.
- Antihistamines on their own are effective for treating the early-phase symptoms of hayfever. First-generation antihistamines reduce rhinorrhoea through their anticholinergic action but do little to relieve the nasal congestion associated with the late-phase response; co-administration of a sympathomimetic decongestant may be helpful.

Topical treatment
Intranasal and ophthalmic preparations are available without prescription for the treatment of hayfever symptoms.

Nasal preparations

Nasal preparations contain anti-inflammatory, sympathomimetic decongestant or antihistamine ingredients.

Anti-inflammatories

- The anti-inflammatory agents available are:
- – beclometasone
- – fluticasone
- – sodium cromoglicate.
- Beclometasone and fluticasone are corticosteroids. They down-regulate the inflammatory response of type I allergic reactions by reducing the number of basophils and mast cells, and by blocking release of mediator substances. They inhibit both early and late responses to allergen exposure, and are therefore effective in relieving nasal congestion.
- Sodium cromoglicate is known as a mast cell stabiliser. Its mode of action is not entirely understood but it is thought to act by stabilising mast cell membranes and preventing their degranulation. It counteracts both the early and late response to allergen exposure.
- Beclometasone, fluticasone and sodium cromoglicate are effective in relieving all nasal symptoms of hayfever. They take some days to achieve optimum effect, and treatment should ideally be started at least 2 weeks before symptoms are expected. Patients should be advised that, if symptoms are already present when treatment is started, it could be several days before an effect is noted and several weeks before full relief is obtained.

Beclometasone and fluticasone

- Beclometasone and fluticasone are presented as aqueous non-aerosol sprays. Absorption from the nasal mucosa is low, and systemic effects are highly unlikely at recommended doses (although pregnant and lactating women are advised to avoid using them unless a doctor regards treatment as essential).
- Any local reactions, such as stinging, burning and aftertaste, are mild and transient.
- Treatment may need to be maintained throughout the hayfever season, and repeated each year. The preparations can be used for up to 3 months without consulting a doctor.
- Beclometasone and fluticasone are licensed for use in adults of 18 years and over.
- They should be avoided if there is infection in the nose or eye. There are otherwise no significant contraindications or interactions.

Sodium cromoglicate

- Sodium cromoglicate is available as a 4% aqueous spray.
- It is a prophylactic agent so treatment should begin before the pollen season starts and continued throughout.

- It is less effective at controlling nasal symptoms than corticosteroids and has the disadvantage of requiring administration at least four times daily. However, it is safe and is suitable for children from 5 years of age.
- There are no specific cautions or contraindications, and it does not interact with other drugs.

Sympathomimetic decongestants
- Drops and sprays containing sympathomimetic decongestants are used to relieve nasal congestion associated with hayfever, and may be useful to begin treatment when the nose is badly blocked.
- Compounds available are:
- oxymetazoline
- phenylephrine
- xylometazoline.
- All exert a rapid and potent vasoconstricting effect when applied directly to the nasal mucosa. They should only be used for short periods as rebound congestion can occur.

Eye preparations
- The agents available are:
- sodium cromoglicate
- lodoxamide
- antihistamine/sympathomimetic decongestant combination.
- Most eye symptoms relating to hayfever will be controlled by oral antihistamines, but if symptoms are persistent or particularly troublesome, eye drops are usually effective.
- Sodium cromoglicate and lodoxamide are mast cell stabilisers. Both are used four times daily and are suitable for children.
- Eye drops are available containing an antihistamine, antazoline sulphate 0.5%, and xylometazoline hydrochloride 0.05%. The latter has vasoconstrictor action and is included as a conjunctival decongestant. This preparation can be used for the short-term treatment of hayfever symptoms, but prolonged use may raise intraocular pressure and precipitate glaucoma. The drops are used twice or three times daily and are suitable for children from 5 years of age.
- All eye drops for allergic conjunctivitis contain the preservative benzalkonium chloride, which is absorbed into soft contact lenses and released onto the cornea during wear, causing inflammation and irritation. Soft lenses should not be worn while using these products; gas-permeable lenses may be inserted 30 minutes after using the eye drops.

Additional advice

- Stay indoors and keep all windows closed (this reduces pollen exposure by a factor of up to 10 000).
- Avoid going out, particularly in the early evening and mid-morning.

- Wear close-fitting sunglasses when outside, and a mask if symptoms are really severe.
- In the car, keep windows closed, especially on motorways. Keep the air-conditioning system on, if there is one.

Self-assessment

Case study

It is mid-summer and you are consulted by a young woman wanting advice about her hayfever. She tells you that she is about 18 weeks pregnant and is experiencing really bad hayfever symptoms. She has been prescribed desloratadine tablets by the obstetrician at the antenatal clinic but they do not relieve all the symptoms. She has a lot of discomfort: her eyes feel very itchy and her nose is permanently blocked. She wants to know if you can recommend anything that might help.

Multiple choice questions
1–3.(Open-book, classification)
Questions 1–3 concern the following drugs available without prescription for the treatment of hayfever symptoms:
a. acrivastine
b. beclometasone
c. cetirizine
d. chlorphenamine
e. fluticasone

Which of the above can be given to children from the age of:
1. 1 year?
2. 6 years?
3. 12 years?

4. (Closed-book, simple completion)
A long-distance lorry driver who has to work every day for the next 5 days asks for something to relieve his hayfever symptoms. Which one of the following antihistamines would be the best to recommend?
a. promethazine
b. diphenhydramine
c. clemastine
d. chlorphenamine
e. cetirizine

Tips

Much of the knowledge and all of the professional decision-making skills you need to answer questions in the registration examination should be acquired through your pre-registration training programme.

chapter 24
Nicotine replacement therapy (NRT)

A range of nicotine replacement products is available to help smokers give up.

Addictive effects of nicotine

- Nicotine is readily absorbed through the oral mucosa and the lungs. Peak blood concentrations are achieved within 30 seconds of a puff of a cigarette.
- The drug acts on the central nervous system, causing transient euphoria, a feeling of relaxation, improved concentration and memory and reduced appetite.
- Withdrawal symptoms are anxiety, difficulty in concentrating and irritability, which are relieved by the next cigarette. Eventually smokers establish a steady blood concentration of nicotine through a regular smoking pattern, preventing withdrawal cravings.
- Psychological and behavioural components contribute to smoking dependence in about equal measure to physiological addiction, and are of two types:
  1. associations that reinforce the habit; they can be positive (e.g. following meals) or negative (e.g. stressful situations)
  2. ritual behaviour associated with lighting, holding and inhaling a cigarette, which the smoker associates with the reward of a dose of nicotine.

Epidemiology

- About 25% of the British population smoke. The number has declined from about 50% in the last 30 years.
- The cost to the National Health Service of treating smoking-related diseases is around £1.7 billion per year.
- One-fifth of all deaths in the UK are the result of smoking-related conditions.
- NRT increases the odds of giving up by 1.5–2 times compared with abstinence alone.

Nicotine replacement therapy

- NRT provides nicotine at a lower level than is obtained through smoking, helping prevent withdrawal symptoms and cravings. After a period at a steady state nicotine intake is progressively reduced to zero, over a total period of 2–3 months.

- Nicotine is efficiently absorbed through the buccal and nasal mucosa, the skin or the lungs from a range of presentations.
- Smokers should stop smoking completely while using any NRT product, although some products are licensed for use for smoking reduction before a quit attempt.
- Different NRT presentations should not be used together.

Presentations

Transdermal patches

- There are two types, both changed daily:
  1. left on for 24 hours, providing a residual nicotine level the next morning that may be better for smokers who crave a cigarette as soon as they wake up
  2. used for 16 hours daily during waking hours only; 24-hour patches can produce sleep disturbances, usually avoided with the 16-hour patch.
- Nicotine plasma concentrations from patches are about half those obtained from smoking the average number of cigarettes per day.
- Patches have the convenience of a once-daily application and may be the most suitable form of NRT for people in whom the behavioural aspect of smoking is relatively unimportant.
- All brands are available in three strengths, providing a smooth reduction in nicotine intake.
- The recommended starting strength is generally the highest, except for light smokers, for whom the medium strength should be used first.
- The recommended treatment period and the length of time on each strength vary between brands, but the overall strategy is a stabilisation period on the high strength for 4–8 weeks, followed by a progressive stepping down of strength over a further 2–8 weeks, before stopping altogether.

Chewing gum

- Nicotine is absorbed from chewing gum through the buccal mucosa.
- Peak blood concentrations are reached in about 2 minutes and the contents of a piece of gum are intended to be released over about 30 minutes.
- A piece of gum is chewed whenever there is an urge to smoke, and it may be the most suitable method for the smoker who finds cigarette cravings difficult to resist. It may also provide a greater sense of control over curbing the habit, and chewing acts as a behavioural substitute for smoking.
- Use of gum mimics the pattern of nicotine intake obtained by smoking, but peak blood levels are lower and the steady-state nicotine concentration is about 30% of that obtained from cigarettes.

Inhalator

- Nicotine is contained in an impregnated porous polyethylene plug inside a plastic tube, and is used in the same way as a cigarette, with puffs taken as desired.

- Each puff delivers about 13 μg nicotine, which is only 4–8% of that obtained per puff of a cigarette. But a plug will last much longer than a cigarette because the available nicotine is released over about 20 minutes, and not only is nicotine intake reduced but the concentration peaks are also flattened.
- Use can be by deep pulmonary inhalation or shallow buccal 'puffing'. Nicotine intake is slightly higher with the former, but both methods produce comparable steady-state plasma concentrations equivalent to those achieved with nicotine gum.
- Recommended use is 6–12 cartridges per day, as required for the first 3 months, after which the daily dosage should be progressively reduced to zero over a further 6–8 weeks.
- The inhalator is intended to address both the physical and behavioural components of smoking cessation, as it involves putting the device to the mouth as in smoking and inhaling 'puffs' as desired. It may be particularly useful for the highly behaviour-dependent smoker.

Sublingual tablets
- Sublingual tablets provide an unobtrusive method of nicotine replacement.
- One sublingual tablet is bioequivalent to one piece of nicotine 2 mg chewing gum, and the recommended dosage is comparable.
- It may be a useful method for smokers who do not like or have difficulty in chewing gum.
- Placed under the tongue, the tablet slowly disintegrates in about 30 minutes.
- Depending on how heavily a person smokes, one or two tablets are used per hour to an absolute maximum of 40 per day. The full dosage should be maintained for 3 months and then gradually reduced to zero within the next 3 months.

Nasal spray
- This provides a fast-acting method of nicotine delivery for highly dependent smokers.
- A 50 μl metered spray, administered to each nostril, delivers a nicotine dose of 1 mg. Nicotine is rapidly absorbed from the nasal mucosa, reaching maximum plasma levels in 10–15 minutes; about half the dose is absorbed.
- One metered spray is inhaled into each nostril when necessary to relieve craving, with a maximum two doses per hour and 64 sprays (32 into each nostril) in 24 hours. As-required dosing can be maintained for up to 8 weeks, after which the dosage should be reduced to zero over the next 4 weeks.
- Side-effects, including nose and throat irritation, watering eyes and coughing, are fairly common, especially in the first couple of weeks.

Lozenges
- As with chewing gum, nicotine is absorbed from lozenges through the buccal mucosa.
- Lozenges provide a more discreet means of NRT than chewing gum, and may be preferred by those who do not like or have difficulty chewing gum, such as denture wearers.

Cautions and contraindications

- NRT products provide much lower doses of nicotine than are obtained by smoking, are free from the toxic effects of tar and carbon monoxide, and can be supplied without prescription to people in the following 'risk' groups:
- – pregnant and breastfeeding women
- – adolescents aged 12–18 years
- – smokers with underlying disease such as cardiovascular, hepatic and renal disease, diabetes mellitus and those taking concurrent medication.
  They should be used with caution in these groups.
- Smokers with any chronic or serious skin condition should avoid patches as there is a possibility of localised skin reactions.
- Nicotine can exacerbate symptoms of peptic ulcer or gastritis, particularly with gum or lozenges, as nicotine may enter the stomach directly.

Adverse effects

- Potential side-effects and withdrawal symptoms from NRT are the same as from smoking, including hiccups, sore throat, headache, nausea and dizziness, but clinical trials have shown most to be comparable with those caused by placebo.
- Transfer of dependence from smoking to NRT products is unlikely, but possible.

Interactions

- Tobacco smoke reduces serum levels of a wide range of drugs and dose adjustment may be necessary when smokers have given up, particularly with theophylline, beta-blockers, adrenergic agonists, nifedipine, tricyclic antidepressants, phenothiazines, benzodiazepines and insulin.

Self-assessment

Case study

One of your regular patients, a heavy smoker who has unsuccessfully tried several times to give up smoking using various NRT products and is currently being treated for depression, asks you what you know about Zyban. He says he has been looking up smoking cures on the internet and found articles on several sites that say Zyban is very effective. He has also had 'spam' e-mails offering it for sale. He wants to know if it is as good as the articles say it is, and if he can buy it from you because he would rather you had the business. How would you respond?

Multiple choice questions

1. (Closed-book, multiple completion)
   To which of the following could nicotine chewing gum be supplied without prescription?
   a. a 14-year-old girl
   b. a 56-year-old man with hypertension
   c. a 20-year-old pregnant woman

2. (Open-book, simple completion)
   Which one of the following is not prescribable on the NHS?
a. Nicobrevin
b. Nicorette inhalator
c. Nicotinell mint 1 mg lozenge
d. Nicotinell mint 2 mg lozenge
e. Niquitin CG 4 mg gum

3–5. (Closed-book, classification)
   Questions 3–5 concern the following NRT products:
a. Nicorette 4 mg gum
b. Nicorette inhalator
c. Nicorette nasal spray
d. Nicorette microtab
e. Nicorette 1 mg lozenge

Which of the above might be the most suitable for:
3. a highly behaviour-dependent smoker?
4. a highly nicotine-dependent smoker?
5. a smoker who finds cravings difficult to resist?

Tips

For calculation questions in the registration exam, it is essential to understand thoroughly and be able to manipulate concentrations expressed in percentages, proportions and parts and as molar quantities.

Skin

Acne	163
Cold sores (oral herpes simplex)	169
Eczema/dermatitis	173
Fungal skin infections	179
Scalp conditions	183

chapter 25
Acne

Acne vulgaris is a common condition in young people. Although it may sometimes be unsightly and can persist for several years, it is not usually serious and resolves in most patients by the age of 25. However, it can have a significant psychological impact as it affects young people at a stage in their lives when they are especially sensitive about their appearance.

Effective treatments for milder forms of acne are available from pharmacies without prescription.

Causes

Acne vulgaris is the result of several factors combined. The condition arises in the pilosebaceous units in the dermis, which consist of a hair follicle and associated sebaceous gland. These glands secrete sebum, a mixture of fats and waxes that protect the skin and hair by retarding water loss and forming a barrier against external agents. The hair follicle is lined with epithelial cells that become keratinised as they mature.

The main processes involved in acne are:
- During puberty the production of androgenic hormones increases in both sexes and testosterone levels rise. Testosterone is taken up into the sebaceous glands where it is converted into dihydrotestosterone, which stimulates the glands to secrete increased sebum.
- At the same time, keratin in the follicular epithelial wall becomes unusually cohesive and sebum accumulates to form keratin plugs. These block the follicle openings in the epidermis and cause them to dilate beneath the skin surface.
- If the orifice of the follicular canal opens sufficiently, the keratinous material extrudes through it and an open comedone results. This is also known as a blackhead, as the keratinous material darkens in contact with the air. Because this material can escape, the comedone does not become inflamed. If the follicular orifice does not open sufficiently, a closed comedone (whitehead) results, within which inflammation can occur. Most acne sufferers have a combination of both.
- Microorganisms, mainly *Propionibacterium acnes*, cause the follicular wall of closed comedones to disrupt and collapse, spilling their contents into the surrounding tissue and provoking an inflammatory response. In addition, bacterial enzymes decompose triglycerides in the sebum to produce free fatty acids, which also cause inflammation. This process leads to the formation of papules around the follicular openings in the more common, milder form of acne and to cyst formation in the deeper layers of the skin in the more severe form.

Epidemiology

- Acne affects approximately 80% of people aged 11–30 years at some time, with about 60% of those sufficiently affected to seek treatment.
- Peak incidence is 14–17 years in females and 16–19 years in males.
- The condition normally resolves within 10 years of onset, but up to 5% of women and 1% of men may suffer into their 30s.
- The incidence of acne appears to have fallen in recent years; the reasons are unknown.

Signs and symptoms

- Distribution: lesions usually occur on the forehead, nose and chin, but the periorbital area is usually spared. In more severe cases, the whole of the face, upper chest and back may be affected.
- Severity: acne vulgaris is classified according to its clinical features:
- Mild: any or all of the following may be present:
  - small, tender, red papules
  - pustules
  - blackheads (small dark plugs of sebum and keratinised epithelial cells)
  - whiteheads (small keratin cysts appearing as white papules).
- Moderate: more frequent papules and pustules, with possibly some scarring
- Severe: nodular abscesses, leading to extensive scarring.

Differential diagnosis

- Rosacea, an inflammatory skin condition causing acne-like papules and pustules. However, there are also redness and flushing of the central facial area and cheeks. The condition usually occurs in young to early middle-aged adults.

Circumstances for referral

- moderate or severe acne
- mild acne, if there is no improvement after 2 months with over-the-counter treatment
- acne beginning or persisting outside the normal age range for the condition (teenage years and early 20s)
- suspected drug-induced acne: acne is a possible side effect of lithium, phenytoin, progestogens, azathioprine and rifampicin
- suspected occupational causes: frequent or prolonged contact with grease and oils may predispose to acne
- suspected rosacea.

Treatment

- Non-prescription topical treatments are usually the first line of treatment for mild to moderate acne. Their overall aim is to remove follicular plugs to allow sebum to flow freely, and to minimise bacterial colonisation of the skin.

Treatments must be used regularly for up to 3 months to produce benefits.
- Types of preparation available are: keratolytics, antimicrobials, anti-inflammatory agents and abrasive products.

Keratolytics

- Keratolytic agents (also known as comedolytics in relation to acne) promote shedding of the keratinised epithelial cells on the skin surface, although the compounds used may do this via different mechanisms.
- Keratolytics prevent closure of the pilosebaceous orifice and the formation of follicular plugs, and facilitate sebum flow. They also possess varying levels of antimicrobial activity, which contribute to their effectiveness.
- The keratolytic compounds in over-the-counter acne products are benzoyl peroxide, salicylic acid, sulphur and resorcinol.

Benzoyl peroxide

- Benzoyl peroxide is generally accepted as the first-line topical treatment for mild to moderate acne.
- It is thought to be both comedolytic, mainly through an irritant effect leading to increased turnover of the follicular epithelial cells and increased sloughing, and bactericidal against *P. acnes*. Benzoyl peroxide is lipophilic and penetrates the follicle well; once absorbed it releases oxygen, which suppresses the bacteria, and reduces the production of irritant free fatty acids.
- Benzoyl peroxide is mildly irritant and may cause redness, stinging and peeling, especially at the start of treatment, but tolerance usually develops with continued use. To minimise these effects, the lowest available strength (usually 5%, but 2.5% is available for highly sensitive skin) should be used and applied at night for the first week so that any erythema subsides by the next morning. If there is no adverse reaction, frequency of application may then be increased to twice daily. Several weeks of regular application are usually required to produce real benefit. If the lower strength is ineffective, the higher strength (10%) can be tried.
- Treatment should not continue beyond 3 months with the 5% preparations or beyond 2 months for 10%. If skin irritation is troublesome the product should be stopped for a day or two, and if there is the same reaction when the product is used again it should be discontinued.
- Care should be taken to keep all keratolytics away from the eyes, mouth and other mucous membranes. Benzoyl peroxide is an oxidising agent and may bleach clothing and bedclothes.
- Benzoyl peroxide is available as creams, lotions, gels and washes (2.5, 5 and 10%, and a 4% cream). There is little difference in clinical response to these concentrations in terms of reducing the number of inflammatory lesions, but formulation appears to make a difference. The drying effect of an alcoholic gel base enhances the effectiveness of the active constituent, and it is more effective than a lotion of the same concentration. However, gels have a greater potential for causing skin dryness and irritation than preparations in aqueous bland bases, so water-based preparations may improve compliance.

Salicylic acid
- Salicylic acid is used in concentrations of up to 2% for acne.
- It exerts its keratolytic effect by increasing the hydration of epithelial cells. It may also have some bacteriostatic activity and a direct anti-inflammatory effect on lesions. It is believed to enhance penetration into the skin of other medicaments, and is combined with sulphur in some formulary preparations.
- Salicylic acid is a mild irritant and similar precautions should be adopted as for benzoyl peroxide. Preparations are applied twice or three times a day. Salicylic acid is readily absorbed through the skin and excreted slowly, and salicylate poisoning can occur if preparations are applied frequently, in large amounts and over large areas. Patients who are sensitive to aspirin should avoid these preparations.

Sulphur and resorcinol
- Sulphur and resorcinol are claimed to possess keratolytic and antiseptic properties, but this is debatable and there is little evidence of effectiveness. Both can cause skin irritation and sensitisation, and resorcinol can cause other adverse effects. Both substances are now little used.

Antimicrobials
- Antimicrobial compounds available in over-the-counter preparations are cetrimide, chlorhexidine, povidone-iodine, triclocarban and triclosan.
- As two of the contributory factors to acne are increased sebum production and *P. acnes*, one approach to treatment is to remove excess sebum from the skin and reduce the bacterial count. To this end, several products are formulated as astringent lotions and detergent-based washes containing antibacterial or antiseptic ingredients, and there are also some antimicrobial creams.

Abrasives
- There is one product containing an abrasive licensed for acne treatment. It contains small, gritty particles in a skin wash, intended to remove follicular plugs mechanically. It is contraindicated in the presence of superficial venules or capillaries (telangiectasia), and overenthusiastic use can cause irritation. There is little evidence of the effectiveness of abrasive preparations in acne.

Anti-inflammatory
- Topical nicotinamide is claimed to have anti-inflammatory activity. It appears to be effective. It may produce side-effects of dryness, peeling and irritation similar to those of benzoyl peroxide, and the same precautions in use should be taken.

Prescription treatments
- Topical comedolytic, antibacterial and combined comedolytic/antimicrobial preparations.

- Oral antibacterials: these can be prescribed if topical therapy alone is ineffective. Tetracycline, oxytetracycline, doxycycline, minocycline, lymecycline, erythromycin and trimethoprim are the agents used. Treatment is long-term – for up to 2 years.
- Hormonal treatment: co-cyprindiol, containing cyproterone, an antiandrogen that decreases sebum production, and ethinylestradiol, can be prescribed for women with moderate to severe acne. It also prevents ovulation and, although it is no more effective for acne than oral antibacterials, it is useful for women who also want oral contraception.
- Oral isotretinoin is available for severe acne refractive to other forms of treatment. It is effective but is teratogenic and can have severe side-effects. It should be prescribed only by, or under the supervision of, a consultant dermatologist.

Additional advice

- There is no evidence that poor hygiene causes acne, but washing the face twice a day with an antibacterial soap or a mild cleanser degreases the skin and removes bacteria, and should help reduce the severity of the condition. Sweat should not be allowed to remain on the skin, but should be washed off as soon as possible.
- Avoid hairstyles in which the hair is constantly touching the face, and shampoo hair regularly.
- Pimples and blackheads should not be squeezed or pinched with the fingers. Comedone expressors (blackhead removers) can be used; removal is aided by exposing the skin to steam first.
- Natural sunlight is thought to be helpful in reducing acne, but overexposure should be avoided.
- Avoid heavy, greasy cosmetics and use water-based moisturisers.
- There is no evidence that fatty foods and chocolate cause acne, but no harm is done by seeing if excluding them from the diet has a beneficial effect.
- A healthy, balanced diet with plenty of water, and regular exercise, is always good advice.

Self-assessment

Case study

A young woman of about 20 asks for your advice on acne. She says that there are times in each month when her skin is perfect and others when she has sudden outbreaks of acne. She says that her mother also suffered in this way and that her acne faded when she started taking an oral contraceptive. She asks if oral contraceptives can be used to treat acne specifically, and if so can she get them over the counter?

Multiple choice questions

1. (Open-book, simple completion)

   A patient wishes to buy a treatment for acne that he has had previously on prescription. Which one of the preparations below could you not sell to him?

a. Differin cream
b. Eskamel cream
c. Nicam gel
d. Panoxyl aquagel 10%
e. Quinoderm cream

2. (Open-book, simple completion)

   Which one of the preparations for acne below could you not dispense against an NHS prescription?

a. Differin cream
b. Eskamel cream
c. Nicam gel
d. Panoxyl aquagel 10%
e. Quinoderm cream

3. (Closed-book, multiple completion)

   A young man asks you for 'something that really works' for his acne. After speaking to him you decide to refer him to his general practitioner. Which of the factors below would lead you to this decision?

a. The young man is 20 years old.
b. He has small, red spots and occasional small, pus-filled spots on his face and upper back.
c. He has already tried two over-the-counter acne preparations for 2 months each.

Tips

In an examination read questions carefully and make sure you understand them before answering. Many marks are lost by candidates who provide an answer that is not relevant to the set question.

chapter 26
Cold sores
(oral herpes simplex)

A cold sore is a painful and unsightly, though not normally serious, recurrent virus infection of the area around the lips.

Causes

- Cold sores are caused by the herpes simplex virus type 1 (HSV-1).
- Transmission of infection is through transfer of the virus via saliva to mucous membranes, e.g. by kissing.
- The infection is usually contracted in childhood; it may not manifest clinically for several years or at all, but the virus is never eliminated from the body.
- Following attacks, the virus regresses to the ganglia of the trigeminal and lumbosacral nerves, where it lies dormant until one of several trigger factors or lowered immunity allows it to break out again.
- Attacks are frequently triggered by the common cold, hence the common name of the condition. Outbreaks also often follow exposure to the sun, giving rise to the other common name, sun blisters.
- Other trigger factors include: fatigue; stress; exposure to cold weather and wind; trauma around the mouth; hormonal changes associated with the menstrual cycle.

Epidemiology

- Cold sores are very common: about 80% of the population are asymptomatic carriers of the virus, and 20–25% of these (about 8 million people) suffer, on average, two symptomatic outbreaks per year.

Signs and symptoms

- Outbreaks may begin with a prodromal phase of up to 24 hours before any visible signs appear, during which the area on or around the lips begins to tingle, burn or itch.
- Erythema then develops, followed by the formation of painful and irritating fluid-filled blisters on the lips and skin around the mouth, which break down into shallow, weeping ulcers within 1–3 days.

- The ulcers dry and form crusts, which are shed, and the area heals within a further 2 weeks.
- The total length of an episode is usually 10–20 days.
- Initial outbreaks in children typically manifest as gingivostomatitis, with lesions all over the inside of the mouth and symptoms of systemic infection. Primary infection in adolescents manifests as pharyngitis, with lesions in the throat and symptoms similar to glandular fever.

Differential diagnosis

- Mouth ulcers: these occur on the mucous membranes and tongue inside the mouth, not on the outside of the lip and mouth.
- Chickenpox: vesicles can occur both around the outside and inside the mouth, but they are also widespread on other parts of the body.
- Impetigo: a bacterial skin infection, more common in children, that usually affects the face but can spread more widely. Lesions are itchy and not confined to the area round the lips, although they may first appear there.
- Lip cancer: lesions develop slowly and are initially painless.
- Primary chancre of syphilis: sores can occur on the lip. A single hard ulcer appears, which is painless, followed by swelling and hardening of lymph glands in the neck, then spreading to lymph glands elsewhere in the body.
- Angular cheilitis: cracks occurring at the corners of the mouth that become inflamed and macerated. It is most common in elderly denture wearers.

Symptoms and circumstances for referral

- young children and babies
- sores that do not heal within 14 days
- painless sores
- multiple sores
- systemic symptoms
- frequent attacks
- any eye involvement. HSV in the eyes can cause herpes simplex keratitis, a potentially sight-threatening infection
- atopic and immunocompromised patients.

Treatment

Cold sores are difficult to treat – even systemic antiviral therapy has not proven particularly effective. Non-prescription treatments are the antiviral agents, aciclovir and penciclovir, and preparations for symptomatic relief containing antiseptics, astringents and local anaesthetics.

Aciclovir
- Aciclovir is presented as a 5% cream.

- Aciclovir is a synthetic analogue of guanine. Its spectrum of activity is specific to human pathogenic viruses that produce thymidine kinase, of which HSV-1 is one.
- Aciclovir is converted by thymidine kinase within viral cells to aciclovir triphosphate, which is then incorporated into viral DNA instead of the deoxyguanosine triphosphate required for DNA synthesis and replication.
- The cream is applied five times daily, at 4-hourly intervals, starting, if possible, as soon as prodromal symptoms occur. Treatment can be continued for up to 10 days, if necessary.
- Evidence of the effectiveness of topical aciclovir has not been convincing, but it may shorten attacks by a day or two if use is begun early enough.
- There is limited evidence that aciclovir cream reduces recurrence of cold sores, but little proof that it protects against attacks caused by ultraviolet radiation, one of the most common triggers of the condition.
- Aciclovir cream is licensed for use in children and pregnant women.

Penciclovir
- Penciclovir is available as 1% cream.
- Its antiviral activity and effectiveness are similar to that of aciclovir.
- It is applied 2-hourly during waking hours.

Other preparations
Products containing combinations of constituents with local anaesthetic and analgesic effects, such as lidocaine, choline salicylate and phenol, counterirritants such as ammonia solution and menthol, and astringents such as zinc sulphate and tannic acid, are marketed to reduce discomfort and promote faster healing of sores while the infection takes its course. Some are formulated with alcoholic bases, which may have a drying effect on sores and speed up healing. The bland cream bases of some products may have a soothing effect.

Combination preparations for cold sores are relatively innocuous. Creams can be applied as frequently as necessary, although lotions and gels are limited to three or four applications per day.

Additional advice

- To prevent spread of infection to the eyes:
- patients should wash their hands after applying treatment
- women should be very careful when applying eye makeup if they have a cold sore.
- To prevent spread of infection to others, people with cold sores should not share towels, face flannels and cutlery with others.
- For sufferers whose attacks are triggered by sunlight, an ultraviolet-blocking lip salve or high-factor sunscreen is an effective prophylactic.

Self-assessment

Case study

A young mother consults you. She says that she feels very guilty because she suffers from cold sores and thinks that she has infected her 4-year-old daughter who has had one attack, brought on by exposure to a cold wind. She wants to know what she can do to prevent her having any more, and to try to prevent her younger son, who is 1 year old, from becoming infected with the virus. What is your advice?

Multiple choice questions

1–3. (Open-book, classification)

Questions 1–3 concern the following medicines:

a. Adcortyl in Orabase
b. Corlan
c. Herpetad
d. Herpid
e. Vectavir

Which of the above:

1. can be prescribed for the treatment of cold sores, but is not recommended?
2. needs to be applied every 2 hours during waking hours for the treatment of cold sores?
3. can be bought without a prescription for the treatment of cold sores?

Tips

In the registration exam open paper the calculation questions are put in a separate section at the end, but it is probably a good idea to tackle them first while you are still fresh.

chapter 27
Eczema/dermatitis

Causes
- The terms 'eczema' and 'dermatitis' are used interchangeably to describe a range of inflammatory skin conditions of which the principal symptoms are dryness, erythema and itch, often with weeping and crusting.
- It has become conventional to apply the term 'eczema' to conditions with an endogenous cause in atopic individuals and 'dermatitis' to reactions to external agents.

Atopic eczema
- Atopic eczema is a chronic fluctuating inflammatory condition of the skin with no known cause, although there is often a genetic link and a family history of allergic sensitivity.

Contact dermatitis
There are two types: irritant and allergic.

Irritant dermatitis
- Irritant dermatitis is the result of direct damage to the skin by a provoking agent on first exposure to a strong irritant, or repeated exposure to a milder one.
- Once the outer keratin layer of the skin has been damaged, irritant substances are able to pass into the cells of the epidermis and cause an inflammatory reaction.
- Irritant agents include: detergents and household cleaning materials; hair tints and perming solutions; building and do-it-yourself materials; and gardening products.
- The condition may be chronic, e.g. from continual wetting of the skin.

Allergic dermatitis
- Allergic dermatitis is the result of hypersensitivity to a sensitising agent.
- It can occur after just a couple of exposures or may take several years of repeated exposure to develop. Once established, sensitivity usually remains for life.
- Sensitising agents include: rubber in household gloves and footwear; nickel in costume jewellery, zips, bra clips and belt buckles; resins in glues; ingredients of cosmetics and toiletries; some plants; paints and cement.

Epidemiology

Eczema

- The incidence of atopic dermatitis is about 3–10% of the population, and appears to be increasing as a result of increase in irritants and pollutants in the home.
- About 50% of patients develop the condition within the first year of life. By age 5, 87% of sufferers have developed their condition. Fewer than 2% develop eczema after the age of 20 years.
- The condition improves with age – about 50% resolve by age 13, and few cases persist beyond the age of 30.

Contact dermatitis

- 85–95% of all occupationally related skin disease in the working population of industrialised countries is due to contact dermatitis.
- In these countries hand dermatitis affects 2–6% of the population.

Signs and symptoms

Atopic eczema

- There is a dry, scaly, often erythematous rash.
- Typical distribution is inside elbows, behind knees and on cheeks, forehead and outer limbs.
- It is very itchy; patients tend to scratch and excoriate the skin, opening the way for bacterial infection. Continued scratching can lead to lichenification (hardened and leathery skin).
- There is usually a family history of atopic disease.
- Patients may have other atopic disease, e.g. asthma, hayfever.
- The disease may be chronic, with periodic acute exacerbations.
- If chronic, the skin will be dry, fissured and painful, and may bleed.

Irritant contact dermatitis

Acute exposure

- Skin is itchy and inflamed, usually red and swollen, and papular with vesicles.
- Lesions develop rapidly within 6–12 hours of contact.
- Distant body sites are not commonly affected.
- Recovery may be rapid if there is no further contact with the irritant.

Chronic exposure

- With chronic exposure there is a dry, irritable, red, scaly eruption.

Allergic contact dermatitis

- There is a history of contact with the allergen.
- In the acute or early stages, the skin is inflamed and itchy with weeping and vesiculation.

- In the chronic stages there is dryness and scaling, with fissuring areas.
- Often there is a sharp cut-off point defined by the area of contact, but in long-standing dermatitis irritation may become generalised and spread to areas not in contact with the allergen.

Differential diagnosis

Common conditions that may have similar features to atopic eczema and contact dermatitis include:
- seborrhoeic dermatitis (see Chapter 29)
- fungal infections (see Chapter 28)
- psoriasis: a chronic skin disease characterised by well-defined dull red, scaly patches
- atopic eczema and contact dermatitis may be confused with each other.

Symptoms and circumstances for referral

- if the condition is severe, with badly fissured or cracked skin and bleeding
- if there is evidence of infection (weeping skin)
- failure of over-the-counter (OTC) treatment
- contact dermatitis with no identifiable cause
- duration longer than 2 weeks.

Treatment

First-line therapy
- moisturisers and emollients (all available OTC)
- corticosteroid creams (some available OTC)
- oral antihistamines (most available OTC).

Second-line therapy
- topical immunosuppressants (tacrolimus, pimecrolimus: prescription-only medicine (POM))
- oral immunosuppressants (corticosteroids; others, e.g. ciclosporin, azathioprine, in specialist secondary care only: POM).

Non-prescription treatments – atopic eczema
Moisturisers and emollients
- Moisturisers and emollients should be used regularly and liberally to keep the skin hydrated. They can be messy to use and time-consuming, but they provide considerable benefit and help prevent flare-ups.
- Eczema is a dry-skin condition, and in general the greasier the preparation, the more moisture-retaining ability it confers on the skin.
- Greasier preparations are better for dry, cracked and thickened skin, and should be applied thickly overnight.
- Thinner creams and lotions rub in more easily and are more cosmetically acceptable, but to be effective need to be reapplied several times a day.

- Emollients should also be used in the bath and as soap substitutes. Emollient topical applications are most effective if applied immediately after a bath, after the skin has been patted dry but still retains some moisture on it.

Corticosteroid creams

- 1% hydrocortisone and 0.05% clobetasone butyrate creams are licensed for pharmacy sale for short-term treatment of mild to moderate eczema.
- Clobetasone is more potent than hydrocortisone and more effective for flare-ups.
- Both are applied sparingly to the affected area(s) twice daily until the condition resolves, for up to a maximum of 7 days.
- There are several licensing restrictions on the use of OTC corticosteroids:
- Application is restricted to 'small areas'.
- OTC corticosteroids may not be used on the face, or in the eyes or anogenital areas.
- They may not be used on ulcerated, broken or weeping skin, or with occlusive dressings.
- They are contrainidicated in pregnancy and during lactation.
- Hydrocortisone is not licensed for use in children under 10.
- Clobetasone may be used in children under 12, on the advice of a doctor.

Oral antihistamines

- Severe pruritus (itching) in children, particularly at night, can be treated with oral antihistamines: chlorphenamine syrup is licensed for use from 1 year, promethazine syrup from 2 years.
- Oral antihistamines can cause drowsiness, although this may be a benefit.

Non-prescription treatments – irritant contact dermatitis

- Topical corticosteroids, if necessary. (They may be used on the earlobes for dermatitis caused by costume jewellery earrings, as this area is not classified as part of the face.)
- Emollients may be used to replace the lipid barrier of the skin.

Non-prescription treatments – allergic contact dermatitis

- Topical corticosteroids if necessary.
- Non-sedating oral antihistamines (acrivastine, cetrizine, loratadine) if necessary; these do not normally cause drowsiness.
- Sedating antihistamines (chlorphenamine, promethazine) can be used for night-time relief of irritable dermatitis.
- (For detail on oral antihistamines, see Chapter 23.)

Additional advice

- In contact dermatitis, try to identify the irritant or allergen and avoid it.
- In atopic eczema, use moisturisers and emollients liberally and often.

■ Eczema sufferers should avoid bubblebath products, soaps and shower gels because they can cause skin sensitisation and excessive dehydration of the skin.

Self-assessment

Case study

A mother brings her 7-year-old daughter to your pharmacy for advice about an itchy rash behind both knees that the girl has had for 3–4 days. In answer to your questions, the mother tells you that her daughter has no rash anywhere else, does not suffer from asthma or hayfever, but does have quite sensitive skin and she has had similar rashes before. On examination, the rash is maculopapular (smooth with some raised lesions) and slightly inflamed. What advice would you give?

Multiple choice questions

1–3. (Closed-book, classification)

Questions 1–3 concern terms for skin lesions that pharmacists should be able to understand and use to other health professionals. The following terms describe different skin lesions:

a. macule
b. nodule
c. papule
d. pustule
e. vesicle

Which of the above, from (a) to (e), are characterised by the following descriptions?

1. a small palpable lesion, usually less than 0.5 cm diameter, raised above the skin surface
2. a smooth area of colour change on the skin less than 1.5 cm diameter
3. a small fluid-filled blister less than 0.5 cm diameter

4. (Closed-book, simple completion)

Which one of the following could be supplied without prescription for treating a 6-year-old child for atopic eczema?

a. betamethasone valerate 0.1% cream
b. clobetasol propionate 0.05% cream
c. clobetasone butyrate 0.05% cream
d. hydrocortisone 0.5% cream
e. hydrocortisone 1% cream

Tips

In multiple choice questions, some distractors are easy to spot and eliminate, narrowing the choice between credible options.

chapter 28
Fungal skin infections

- Topical fungal infections are mostly caused by dermatophytes, organisms that invade and proliferate on the outermost, horny layer (stratum corneum) of the skin, hair and nails.
- They do not normally penetrate deeper into the skin or tissues. They tend to thrive in areas of the body that are occluded and moist.
- The common infecting organisms are *Trichophyton*, *Microsporum* and *Epidermophyton* species.
- Common fungal skin infections for which pharmacists can provide advice and treatment include:
- tinea pedis (athlete's foot: see Chapter 7)
- tinea corporis (ringworm)
- tinea cruris (dhobie itch, jock itch).
- Pityriasis versicolor, a superficial skin infection caused by a yeast, *Pityrosporum orbiculare* (also known as *Malassezzia furfur*), can be treated with similar non-prescription preparations to fungal infections.

Tinea corporis (ringworm)
Causes and epidemiology

- Tinea corporis is a fungal infection of the major skin surfaces, excluding the feet, face, hands, groin and scalp.
- It is often transmitted by animals (pets or livestock) and can also be picked up from the soil.
- Children are particularly susceptible and can easily pass it on to other children. Adults can also become infected. Farmers and people who work with furry animals are at increased risk.

Signs and symptoms

- There are itchy pink or red scaly patches with a well-defined inflamed border.
- Lesions are often paler at the centre, becoming progressively inflamed towards the outer edge.
- Lesions often occur singly, but can be multiple and sometimes overlap to form a large continuous patch.

Differential diagnosis

- Discoid eczema – lesions of similar shape to ringworm, but larger and mainly occurring on the arms, legs, hands and feet. The condition is rare in patients under 20 years.

- Erythrasma – a bacterial infection. Lesions are wrinkled, slightly scaly, and pink, brown or macerated white. They usually occur in the axillae and groins or between toes, and usually do not itch.
- Psoriasis – raised, erythematous and scaly lesions, salmon pink or full rich red in colour, with a surface silvery scale. Lesions appear particularly on the scalp and sacral area, and over the extensor aspect of the knees and elbows.

Symptoms and circumstances for referral

Refer if any of the above conditions is suspected, or if diagnosis is uncertain.

Treatment

- an imidazole cream or terbinafine cream or gel (for details, see Chapter 7).

Additional advice

To prevent reinfection, particularly in children:
- Avoid close contact with pets and farm animals.
- Wash skin areas that have been in contact with pets and farm animals as soon as possible afterwards.
- Avoid touching or sharing towels with an infected person.

Tinea cruris (dhobie itch, jock itch)
Causes and epidemiology

Tinea cruris is a fungal infection of the groin, occurring almost exclusively in young men.

Signs and symptoms

- There is a brownish-red itchy rash, with a well-defined border, in the groin.
- Infection often spreads to involve the lower abdomen, scrotum and buttocks.

Differential diagnosis and circumstances for referral

- Contact dermatitis, possibly caused by detergents used for washing underwear, may be confused with tinea cruris. It is important to diagnose accurately, as management of the conditions is different.
- The condition may also be confused with erythrasma (see above).

Treatment

Treatment is as for tinea corporis.

Additional advice

To prevent reinfection:

- Wash and thoroughly dry the groin area daily.
- Change underwear daily.
- Do not share towels with others.

Pityriasis versicolor
Epidemiology

- The organism is more common in hot, sunny areas.
- Incidence has increased in recent years with increased travel to subtropical and tropical regions, and warmer summers in the UK.

Signs and symptoms

- Macular (flat) patches of altered pigmentation occurring mainly on the trunk and upper legs and arms.
- In white-skinned people patches are brownish and look as if suntanned, whereas on darker-skinned or heavily tanned people patches are pale or white. The affected area has an overall dappled appearance.
- There is a superficial scale that can be removed by scraping with a fingernail.
- Pruritus, if any, is mild.

Differential diagnosis and circumstances for referral

The condition is most likely to be confused with vitiligo, but vitiligo is much more widespread over the body and usually includes the face.

Treatment

- an imidazole cream applied daily for 3 weeks
- ketoconazole 2% shampoo. Apply undiluted and wash off after 5 minutes. Repeat daily for 1 week, then weekly for several weeks to prevent reinfection.
- selenium sulphide shampoo (unlicensed indication). Apply undiluted and wash off after 4–5 hours. Use weekly for 8 weeks.

Additional advice

To prevent reinfection, ketoconazole shampoo should be used as above once a fortnight.

Self-assessment

Case study

A man in his mid-20s asks for something to clear up a skin condition that he has had for several months since returning from a holiday in Thailand. In response to your questions it emerges that the condition started with uneven, scaly patches on his upper chest where the skin didn't tan when he sunbathed. The patches have since spread to his entire back, chest and abdomen. He describes his skin as looking like a snake's and says he can scrape off the scales with his fingernail. The patches were not itchy to start with but are now. He saw his general practitioner about it and was prescribed an emollient cream that has not made any difference. Could you offer any advice?

Multiple choice questions

1–3. (Closed-book, classification)

Questions 1–3 concern the following topical fungal infections:

a.   tinea capitis
b.   tinea corporis
c.   tinea cruris
d.   tinea pedis
e.   tinea unguium

Which of the above conditions:

1.   characteristically occurs on the face and neck?
2.   characteristically occurs in the groin?
3.   characteristically occurs between the toes?

4.   (Open-book, assertion/reason)
     You receive the following FP10NC (England) prescription (WP10NC in Wales, GP10 in Scotland):

(Patient's name, address and age)

The body of the prescription reads:

4 × 30 g Nizoral cream

Apply daily for pityriasis versicolor, until 2 weeks after the condition has cleared.

(Date of prescribing and prescriber's signature)

First statement: This prescription should not be dispensed.
Second statement: Nizoral cream is not prescribable on the NHS; it must be prescribed generically as 'ketoconazole cream'.

Tips

If you feel ill or experience some adverse event during the registration examination, report it to an invigilator and follow up with documentary evidence to the Royal Pharmaceutical Society immediately afterwards. If you wait to see if you have failed before reporting illness, you are very unlikely to receive any consideration from the examiners.

chapter 29
Scalp conditions

This chapter covers the common scalp conditions that pharmacists are likely to encounter: dandruff (pityriasis capitis), seborrhoeic dermatitis, cradle cap, scalp psoriasis and scalp ringworm (tinea capitis). Head lice, another common scalp problem, is covered in Chapter 17.

Dandruff
Causes

- Dandruff (pityriasis capitis) is a chronic, non-inflammatory condition due to a naturally increased rate of horny substance production and cell turnover on the scalp.
- It is now generally recognised to be associated with the presence of high levels of the yeast *Pityrosporum ovale*, although it has not been determined conclusively whether the yeast is the cause of the condition or merely encouraged by the abundance of nutrients from shed skin cells.
- It may also be associated with raised androgen levels.

Epidemiology

- Dandruff is rare in young children, but incidence increases rapidly and reaches its peak in the second decade of life, declining gradually thereafter.
- Estimates of prevalence vary from between 75 and 97% of the population being affected at some time in their lives.
- Both sexes are affected equally.

Signs and symptoms

- excessive shedding of dead skin cells of the scalp in the form of scales, sometimes accompanied by itching and redness.

Differential diagnosis

- All the conditions discussed in this chapter, except tinea capitis, share common signs and can be confused with each other.
- For mild cases this does not usually matter as the conditions can all be controlled with similar over-the-counter (OTC) medications. But care must be taken with more severe manifestations and patients should be referred in any case of doubt.

Symptoms and circumstances for referral

- dandruff persisting or becoming more severe despite treatment
- scaling also affecting other parts of the body, indicating the possibility of seborrhoeic dermatitis, eczema or psoriasis
- a sudden strong tendency to flaking or seborrhoeic dermatitis for the first time in a middle-aged person may be a sign of human immunodeficiency virus (HIV) infection.

Treatment

- Topical treatments for dandruff and mild forms of seborrhoeic dermatitis are the same.
- Regular use (at least twice weekly) of an ordinary mild detergent shampoo will effectively control dandruff by removing scales.
- A wide range of medicated treatments is available, containing:
- pyrithione zinc
- selenium sulphide
- ketoconazole
- coal tar
- salicylic acid.

Pyrithione zinc and selenium sulphide

- Both compounds are cytostatic agents, and act by reducing the rate of epidermal cell turnover. They are generally accepted as being effective in controlling dandruff.
- Pyrithione zinc's action is thought to be due to a non-specific toxicity for epidermal cells; selenium sulphide is believed to have a direct antimitotic effect.
- Both are used as shampoos.
- Pyrithione zinc is used twice or three times weekly, and each application is left on the hair for 2–3 minutes before being rinsed off.
- Selenium sulphide is used twice weekly for 2 weeks, then weekly as necessary. Two applications per treatment should be used, and each left on the hair for 3 minutes.
- Both pyrithione zinc and selenium sulphide are safe for long-term use but selenium sulphide is highly toxic if ingested orally.
- Regular use of selenium sulphide shampoo tends to leave a residual odour of hydrogen sulphide and makes the scalp oily; the hair should not be dyed or permed for at least 2 days either side of using the product.
- Rare contact dermatitis and hypersensitivity are possible with both compounds. Neither compound should be applied to broken or abraded skin and contact with the eyes should be avoided.
- Neither compound is contraindicated in pregnancy or breastfeeding, but selenium sulphide should not be used during the first trimester of pregnancy.
- Selenium sulphide shampoo is not recommended for use in children under 5 years.

- Pyrithione zinc is available in several proprietary and own brands of antidandruff shampoos, which are not licensed as medicines.

Ketoconazole
- Ketoconazole is available as a 2% shampoo.
- It is an azole antifungal that inhibits replication of yeast cells by interfering with the synthesis of ergosterol – a vital component of the cell membrane.
- It is effective in clearing dandruff and scalp seborrhoea.
- To clear dandruff and seborrhoeic dermatitis, the shampoo is used twice weekly for 2–4 weeks, and each application is left on the hair for 3–5 minutes. The condition can then be controlled with weekly or fortnightly use.
- Ketoconazole shampoo appears to be very safe to use. Skin irritation has been reported only very rarely. Ketoconazole is not contraindicated in pregnancy.

Coal tar
- The mode of action of coal tar is unknown but it appears to prevent the formation of dandruff flakes by interfering with the formation of the intracellular 'cement' that holds the discarded dead skin cells together.
- It also appears to inhibit the production of sebum and to have antipruritic properties, making it useful in the treatment of seborrhoeic dermatitis (see below).
- A wide range of shampoos and scalp lotions containing coal tar is available.

Salicylic acid
- Salicylic acid is a keratolytic agent that loosens and sloughs off dead skin cells from the scalp.
- Shampoo formulations may be diluted in use below an effective level and contact time with the scalp may be too short to be effective.
- Ointment preparations containing salicylic acid and coal tar are also available; these are likely to be more effective than shampoos but can be messy to use and the risk of irritation is greater.

Seborrhoeic dermatitis
Causes

- Seborrhoeic dermatitis (seborrhoea) is the result of accelerated skin cell growth and sebaceous gland activity on the scalp, face and trunk. The condition may also involve the area in and around the ears, the eyebrows and eyelashes.
- As in dandruff, *P. ovale* may be a causative agent.

Epidemiology

- Seborrhoeic dermatitis is common in infants, when it is known as cradle cap (see below), relatively rare in children and occurs again from puberty, reaching its peak incidence between the ages of 18 and 40.

Signs and symptoms

- On the scalp, the condition may be difficult to distinguish from more severe forms of dandruff, as characteristic features are the presence of greasy scales and often pruritus.

Differential diagnosis

See under Dandruff, above.

Symptoms and circumstances for referral

- The condition may be difficult to differentiate from scalp psoriasis (see below).
- Severe seborrhoeic dermatitis requires diagnosis and management by a doctor. It is characterised by persistent greasy yellow scales extending over part of the face, the eyebrows and creases on either side of the nose. It may extend to the centre of the back, the chest, the armpits and groin.

Treatment

Treatment is as for dandruff (see above).

Cradle cap
Causes

- Cradle cap is a form of seborrhoeic dermatitis of the scalp in infants, causing scaling and crusting.
- It usually appears within the first 3 months of life and resolves spontaneously within a year.

Signs and symptoms

- Cradle cap appears as scaling and crusting of the scalp in infants.
- Its appearance may be worrying to parents, but the baby is usually happy and not troubled and the condition is usually not serious.

Symptoms and circumstances for referral

Acute, erythematous scaling of scalp, nappy area, face, chest, back and limb flexures may indicate generalised infantile seborrhoeic dermatitis. Atopic eczema is also a possibility.

Treatment

- The *British National Formulary* recommends applications of olive oil or arachis oil, followed by shampooing.

- Proprietary shampoos and creams containing salicylic acid, coal tar or mild detergents are available, but are probably no more effective.

Scalp psoriasis
Causes

Psoriasis is a chronic skin disease characterised by inflammation of the skin and hyperproliferation of skin cells.

Epidemiology

- Scalp psoriasis affects about 3% of the population and both sexes equally.
- Onset is most common between 15 and 40 years of age, and is rare under 10 years.

Signs and symptoms

- Lesions are characteristically well defined, raised, erythematous and scaly, and salmon pink or full rich red in colour.
- There is a surface silvery scale which may be easily removed, often leading to pinpoint capillary bleeding.
- There may be itching, but this is not usually a prominent feature.
- Scalp psoriasis often extends just below the scalp margin, leaving an inflamed, scaly border.

Symptoms and circumstances for referral

Patients with moderate to severe psoriasis may require treatment under the supervision of a dermatologist.

Treatment

- tar-based shampoos and salicylic acid preparations, but they should only be used under medical supervision
- potent topical steroid or calcipitriol preparations (prescription-only medicines (POM)).

Scalp ringworm (tinea capitis)
Causes

Tinea capitis is a fungal infection of the scalp that is often acquired from cats and dogs.

Epidemiology

Scalp ringworm occurs almost exclusively in children.

Signs and symptoms

- round, scaly, bald patches with broken hairs around them
- there is little or no itching.

Symptoms and circumstances for referral

- In severe cases a kerion, a swollen mass discharging pus, will appear on the scalp. It may become inflamed and painful.
- Severe alopecia may develop.
- Secondary bacterial infection can occur.
- The lymph nodes of the neck may also become swollen and tender, and in rare cases there may also be a fever.

Treatment

Treatment with prescription-only systemic antifungals (e.g. griseofulvin) is necessary. No OTC treatments are available.

Self-assessment

Case study

A young man asks you for advice about his severe dandruff, which seems to be getting worse. It is not itchy but it is extremely flaky and embarrassing. He has tried various antidandruff shampoos and nothing seems to work. He asks if there is any cure.

Multiple choice questions

1. (Closed-book, simple completion)

    For which one of the following scalp conditions is there no non-prescription treatment available?

   a. *Pediculus humanus capitis infection*
   b. pityriasis capitis
   c. scalp psoriasis
   d. seborrhoeic dermatitis
   e. tinea capitis

2–4. (Closed-book, classification)

    Questions 2–4 relate to the following scalp conditions:

   a. *Pediculus humanus capitis* infection
   b. pityriasis capitis
   c. scalp psoriasis
   d. seborrhoeic dermatitis
   e. tinea capitis

    For which of the above conditions are the symptoms or signs described below characteristic?

2. round, scaly, bald patches with broken hairs around them

3. well-defined, raised, erythematous and scaly lesions, salmon pink or full rich red in colour
4. a silvery scale on the surface of the scalp which can be easily removed, often leading to pinpoint capillary bleeding

Tips

In the open-book paper of the registration exam, save time by not looking up questions to which you think you know the answers. If you have time at the end of the exam, you can then check answers in the reference texts.

Women's conditions

Cystitis	193
Dysmenorrhoea	197
Emergency hormonal contraception (EHC)	203
Premenstrual syndrome (PMS)	207
Vaginal thrush	211

chapter 30
Cystitis

Causes

Cystitis is an inflammation of the bladder and urethra. Microbial infection is the cause in about half of all cases. The female urethra is very short (about 3 cm) and infecting organisms are readily transferred from the perineum and anus to the bladder.

Epidemiology

- Cystitis is very common in women, affecting over 2 million per year and 50% of women have at least one attack in their lifetime.
- Urethral syndrome, which affects 20–30% of adult women and may have one of several functional or psychogenic causes, has similar symptoms to cystitis caused by infection (lower urinary tract infection).
- Cystitis is uncommon in young men; as well as the urethra being longer than in women, prostatic fluid is thought to possess antibacterial properties. Cystitis is more frequent in older men, where it may be due to prostatic disease or bladder neoplasms.
- Cystitis is uncommon in children.

Signs and symptoms

- abrupt onset; attacks often begin with an itching or pricking sensation in the urethra
- frequent desire to urinate, although only a few drops may be passed
- dysuria – burning or stinging when passing water
- urine may be dark and cloudy, and have an unpleasant 'fishy' odour
- may be raised temperature or fever
- may be pain in the suprapubic area or lower back.

Differential diagnosis

- Pyelonephritis: infection of the upper urinary tract – ureter and kidney. Patients will generally have loin pain (i.e. in the back at about the level of the kidneys) and symptoms of a systemic infection.
- Sexually transmitted diseases, particularly *Chlamydia* and gonorrhoea. Symptoms develop more slowly and persist for longer than with cystitis. There is usually also pus in the urine, making it cloudy and foul-smelling.
- Parasitic infection – schistosomiasis and bilharzia – usually contracted in the

Middle East or North Africa. If suspected, pharmacists should ask about recent foreign travel.
- Oestrogen deficiency in postmenopausal women. This leads to thinning of the endometrial tissue with increased susceptibility to irritation and trauma and cystitis-like symptoms. It can be corrected by hormone replacement or topical oestrogen therapy. Vaginal lubricants can be used if symptoms are caused by intercourse. 'Honeymoon' cystitis may occur in younger women as a consequence of increased sexual activity.
- Contact dermatitis caused by use of bath additives and vaginal deodorants.

Symptoms and circumstances for referral

- all males
- pregnant women
- children
- haematuria (although this does not necessarily have serious implications)
- vaginal discharge (indicates vaginal infection of fungal or bacterial origin)
- loin pain and tenderness (may indicate infection in the kidneys or ureters)
- fever
- symptoms persisting for more than 2 days
- recurrent attacks.

Treatment

Symptomatic
- dilution of urine and 'flushing through' of any causative organisms by drinking large quantities of fluids – water, soft drinks and barley water
- alkalinisation of acidic urine, which causes irritation, with over-the-counter preparations.

Alkalinising agents
- Alkalinising agents are the only treatments available specifically for cystitis without prescription.
- They act by neutralising the urine which becomes acidic, particularly when there is bacterial infection, causing irritation of the bladder.
- Preparations contain either sodium or potassium citrate or sodium carbonate. They are supplied as 2-day courses of single-dose sachets, taken three times daily in a large glass of water.
- A formulary preparation, Potassium Citrate Mixture BP, is also available; it is as effective as other preparations but is less palatable.
- Sodium bicarbonate, 3 g (a level teaspoonful) in water every 2 hours until symptoms subside, can also be used.
- If symptoms persist after 2 days of treatment the patient should be referred to a doctor.
- Cautions:
- Sodium-containing preparations can lead to fluid retention and raised blood pressure and should be avoided in patients with hypertension, cardiovascular

disease, diabetes and impaired renal function and during pregnancy. They should also be avoided by patients taking lithium, as the effectiveness of lithium may be reduced.
- There is a theoretical risk of hyperkalaemia with preparations containing potassium citrate. Such preparations should be avoided in patients taking potassium-sparing diuretics, spironolactone and angiotensin-converting enzyme inhibitors, and in patients with heart or kidney disease.
- Paracetamol or ibuprofen can be used to relieve pain and reduce temperature.

Antibacterials
- A short course of trimethoprim, amoxicillin or nitrofurantoin can be prescribed.
- An application has been made for the reclassification of trimethoprim from prescription-only medicine (POM) to P status, but no product is yet available.

Additional advice

To reduce the possibility of attacks:
- Void the bladder completely when urinating: wait for 20 seconds once the bladder feels empty, then strain to squeeze out the final drops.
- Avoid delay in emptying the bladder; pass water at least every 3 hours.
- After bowel motions, wipe from front to back to minimise transfer of faecal organisms to the vagina and urethra.
- Cystitis is often associated with sexual intercourse. If this seems to be a trigger, wash the perianal skin beforehand and empty the bladder before and after. Use a lubricant to prevent trauma and soreness.
- Avoid tight underwear made from synthetic materials and tight trousers. Thoroughly rinse out detergent after washing clothes.
- Avoid perfumed bath additives and vaginal deodorants, as they may be irritant.
- Reduce intake of coffee and alcohol as these act as bladder irritants in some people.
- There is evidence that drinking cranberry juice regularly (300 ml/day) is prophylactic.

Self-assessment

Case study

A young woman is referred to you by your medicines counter assistant, as she has picked up a General Sales List alkalinising treatment for cystitis but she tells your assistant she has not used such a product before. The client says that she thinks she has cystitis, but when you ask her if she has had cystitis before she says no, but she has talked about her symptoms to a friend who has had cystitis, and her friend thinks that this is what it is. In response to your questions, the symptoms she describes are: urine not being passed more frequently than normal, but dark with an unpleasant smell; pain about halfway up her back on both sides, and she has been feeling feverish since she woke up this morning.

Would you sell the alkalinising treatment to the woman? If not, what would you do or recommend?

Multiple choice questions

1. (Closed-book, simple completion)
   For which one of the following might you be able to recommend an over-the-counter treatment for cystitis?
   a. a 25-year-old man feeling like he wants to pass urine every few minutes, but passing very little with a stinging sensation when he does, and no other symptoms
   b. a 25-year-old woman feeling like she wants to pass urine every few minutes, but passing very little with a stinging sensation when she does, and no other symptoms, returning for the third time in 3 weeks
   c. a 45-year-old woman feeling like she wants to pass urine every few minutes, but passing very little with a stinging sensation when she does, and no other symptoms
   d. a 25-year-old woman passing dark-coloured urine at normal frequency with a burning sensation, and no other symptoms
   e. a 10-year-old girl feeling like she wants to pass urine every few minutes, but passing very little with a stinging sensation when she does, and no other symptoms

2. (Open-book, classification)
   Which of the following could be recommended for over-the-counter treatment of cystitis?
   a. Cymalon sachets
   b. Potassium Citrate Mixture BP
   c trimethoprim 200 mg tablets

3. (Closed-book, assertion/reason)
   First statement: Alkalinising agents containing sodium or potassium salts should not be sold to patients taking drugs for hypertension.
   Second statement: Alkalinising agents containing sodium or potassium salts may cause fluid retention and raise blood pressure.

Tips

For exams, try to memorise the four or five most important symptoms and referral factors for each minor ailment.

chapter 31
Dysmenorrhoea

- Primary dysmenorrhoea (PD) describes painful menstruation in the absence of detectable pelvic pathology. It generally starts a year or so after menarche (the first period), once ovulatory cycles are established. Peak incidence is between 15 and 25 years of age, and then declines with age. It can often be treated with over-the-counter (OTC) medication.
- Secondary dysmenorrhoea (SD) describes painful menstruation attributed to pelvic pathology. It is uncommon before the age of 25 years. Referral is necessary if SD is suspected.

The main features of PD and distinguishing features from SD are described below.

Causes

The cause of PD is thought to be increased uterine activity. This may result from:
- overproduction of prostaglandins, which cause the contractions that shed and expel the endometrium together with the unfertilised ovum
- increased sensitivity of endometrial muscle to prostaglandins.

Other possible causative factors are:
- ischaemia – increased contraction of the myometrium may reduce blood flow, causing 'uterine angina' and crampy pain
- increased production of vasopressin, which increases both the synthesis of prostaglandins and myometrial activity.

Epidemiology

- Estimates of prevalence of PD in young women range from 45 to 95%.
- 5–20% of young women report that PD is so bad that it interferes with normal daily activities.

Signs and symptoms

See Table 31.1 for distinguishing features of PD and SD.

Differential diagnosis

Common possible causes of SD include:
- Endometriosis: the most common cause of SD. Fragments of endometrial tissue become detached, find their way and adhere to abdominal and pelvic structures outside the uterus. Each piece undergoes the monthly cycle of thickening, shedding and bleeding, causing severe pain.

Table 31.1 Main distinguishing clinical features of primary and secondary dysmenorrhoea

Feature	Possible indication	
	Primary dysmenorrhoea	**Secondary dysmenorrhoea**
Age	Under 25 years	Over 25–30
Nature of pain	Crampy, colicky pain in the lower abdomen; may radiate to the back of the legs or the lower back	Dull, continuous, diffuse abdominal pain
Onset of pain	Within a day or two before start of bleeding, until within a day or two after	Several days before start of bleeding and continuing for several days after
Relation to having had children	Before birth of first child	After birth of first child
Vaginal discharge	No discharge	Discharge (may indicate pelvic infection)
Associated symptoms	Nausea, vomiting, gastrointestinal discomfort, constipation, headache, backache, fatigue, faintness, dizziness	Backache, fatigue, menorrhagia (heavy periods), dyspareunia (painful intercourse)

- Mittelschmerz: some women experience mid-cycle pain when ovulation occurs. This is normal, but in some cases the pain is very severe and the cycle is shortened, with mid-cycle pain immediately followed by premenstrual and then menstrual pain.
- Pelvic inflammatory disease (PID): acute pelvic infection occurs when infection occurs in the fallopian tube. Pain is severe and accompanied by fever and discharge. Chronic PID can follow from an acute infection, causing less severe pain associated with menstruation. Sexual intercourse may be painful.
- Intrauterine devices, as well as sometimes causing discomfort and heavier periods, can also cause infection.
- Fibroids (fibromyomas): benign smooth-muscle tumours of the uterus. They are common in women over 40, about 20% of whom have them. They are often symptomless but can cause severe pain associated with menstruation and heavy menstrual bleeding. They are oestrogen-dependent and shrink down after the menopause.

Symptoms and circumstances for referral

- women over 30
- abnormal bleeding
- abnormal vaginal discharge
- fever
- pain extending beyond 48 hours either side of start of menstruation
- pain worsening after start of menstruation
- severe mittelschmerz and bleeding
- pain with a late period (possibility of ectopic pregnancy)
- pain unresponsive to OTC treatment.

Treatment

- Few OTC treatments are licensed and promoted specifically for PD, but many analgesic products list PD as an indication.
- Analgesic preparations are all based on one of three drugs – aspirin, paracetamol and ibuprofen – sometimes in combination with the ancillary analgesics codeine or dihydrocodeine, or with other constituents that are claimed to increase effectiveness. (Author's note: please check and amend at proof stage: An application has been made for P classification for naproxen for PD, and it may be reclassified before the book is published.)

Aspirin, ibuprofen and paracetamol

- Aspirin and ibuprofen are non-steroidal anti-inflammatory drugs (NSAIDs) that exert their therapeutic action by interfering with the biosynthesis of prostaglandins, which are major contributors to inflammation and pain.
- NSAIDs act by blocking the enzyme cyclo-oxygenase, thus preventing the formation of prostaglandin endoperoxides from arachidonic acid produced when tissue is damaged. The action of NSAIDs is therefore local at the site of tissue damage and inflammation, and theoretically they should be more effective for dysmenorrhoea than paracetamol or opioid analgesics, which act centrally.
- The mechanism of action of paracetamol is not well understood; it has little anti-inflammatory activity but is an effective analgesic and antipyretic. Its activity may be due to selective inhibition of cyclo-oxygenase in the central nervous system rather than in peripheral tissues, but there is evidence that paracetamol also acts peripherally at pain chemoreceptors.

Aspirin

- Because of its more pronounced adverse reaction profile, aspirin has now been largely superseded in proprietary products in favour of paracetamol and ibuprofen.
- Adverse drug reactions relevant to girls and women likely to be using aspirin for PD include:
- gastric irritation and bleeding
- hypersensitivity reactions, provoking asthma attacks, urticaria and angioedema.
- Aspirin is also associated with Reye's syndrome, a rare but potentially fatal encephalopathy of infants and children, and it is not licensed for use in children under the age of 16.

Ibuprofen

- Ibuprofen may also cause gastric side-effects, although they are generally less serious than with aspirin.
- Hypersensitivity reactions are also less likely, no interaction normally occurs with anticoagulants in normal doses, and there is no association with Reye's syndrome.

Paracetamol

- Paracetamol is generally safe, its only major drawback being its hepatotoxicity in overdose. Paracetamol is metabolised in the liver where it is converted to a highly reactive toxic intermediate, which is normally detoxified by conjugation with glutathione. In overdose this detoxification mechanism is overwhelmed. The free toxic metabolite then combines with hepatic macromolecules causing hepatitis and necrosis, which often proves fatal. The toxic level of paracetamol need not be greatly above the therapeutic level (4 g daily for adults and children over 12 years) and symptoms of overdose may not appear for 2 days or more. It is therefore extremely important to ensure that patients do not exceed the recommended dosage or use more than one product containing paracetamol at a time.

Ancillary analgesics

Opioids

- Codeine and dihydrocodeine are weak narcotic opioid analgesics useful for the treatment of mild to moderate pain.
- They act directly on opiate receptors in the brain producing analgesia, and also respiratory depression, euphoria and sedation, although these are not usually a problem at OTC doses.
- At non-prescription dosage levels the major side-effect is constipation.
- Codeine is combined with paracetamol in co-codamol tablets and with aspirin in co-codaprin tablets.
- There are also several proprietary preparations combining paracetamol or ibuprofen with codeine, and a paracetamol/dihydrocodeine combination (non-proprietary co-dydramol tablets contain a higher dose of dihydrocodeine and are prescription-only (POM)).

Caffeine

- Several OTC analgesic preparations contain caffeine, the rationale being that as a central nervous system stimulant caffeine will alleviate the depression often associated with pain.
- It has also been claimed that caffeine facilitates absorption of analgesics and enhances their action, but this is disputed.
- Caffeine is habit-forming, can add to gastrointestinal adverse effects and may itself induce headache in large doses or on withdrawal.

Other constituents

- Some analgesic preparations also contain sedating antihistamines, such as diphenhydramine and doxylamine, for their claimed sedative and muscle-relaxant effects.
- They may also have some value as antiemetics in patients who experience nausea or vomiting among their dysmenorrhoea symptoms.

Additional advice

- Symptomatic treatment with a warm bath or locally applied heat (such as hot-water bottle) may provide relief.

- Exercise decreases the severity of menstrual cramps through generation of endorphins, 'the body's own painkillers'.
- Avoid smoking, as this has been associated with increased menstrual pain and heavier bleeding.

Self-assessment

Case study

A teenage girl asks if she can discuss something with you in private. You take her to the consultation area. Once there, she tells you that she has started to get crampy abdominal pains around the start of her periods and wants to know if you can recommend any effective treatment. In response to your questions she tell you she is 16, has been having periods since she was 13, but they have been getting painful in the last few months. The pains usually begin about 12 hours before a period starts and have gone by about 12 hours afterwards, but they can be very painful while they last. Her periods have always been regular and there has been no change in regularity lately. She has tried paracetamol tablets, which have helped a bit, but wonders if there is anything better. Can you recommend treatment in this case, and what would you recommend?

Multiple choice questions

1. (Open-book, multiple completion)
   Which of the following drugs are indicated for the treatment of dysmenorrhoea and can be sold without prescription?
a. ibuprofen
b. alverine citrate
c. diflunisal

2. (Closed-book, multiple completion)
   A woman asks you to recommend something for period pains. Which of the following information that she gives you would make you decide that she should be referred to a doctor?
a. The pain is crampy and colicky, in the lower abdomen and radiating down the back of her legs.
b. The pains start about a day before the start of bleeding and last until about a day after.
c. She is 35 years old.

3. (Closed-book, assertion/reason)
   First statement: Aspirin and ibuprofen are non-steroidal anti-inflammatory drugs (NSAIDs) and theoretically the best OTC analgesics for dysmenorrhoea.
   Second statement: NSAIDs act by promoting the action of the enzyme cyclo-oxygenase, thus preventing the formation of prostaglandin endoperoxides from arachidonic acid produced when tissue is damaged.

Tips

In multiple choice question examinations, watch out carefully for negatives in questions.

chapter 32
Emergency hormonal contraception (EHC)

- Levonorgestrel was reclassified for pharmacy sale in 2001 for EHC (also known as 'the morning-after pill') for women of 16 years and over.
- It is available as a 1500 µg single-dose tablet.
- Schemes operated in some areas by National Health Service primary care organisations permit pharmacists to supply EHC in accordance with patient group directions to girls under 16.

Mode of action

- Levonorgestrel is thought to act in one of several ways, depending on the point in the menstrual cycle at which it is used:
- Before ovulation it may prevent ovulation by delaying or inhibiting the release of the ovum from the ovary.
- After ovulation it may prevent fertilisation by affecting the motility of the fallopian tube and preventing sperm from meeting the ovum.
- After fertilisation it induces changes in the endometrium that render it unreceptive to the ovum and prevent implantation.
- All mechanisms are considered to be contraceptive rather than abortifacient, as clinically conception and the start of the pregnancy are not considered to have occurred until a fertilised ovum is implanted in the endometrium.

Efficacy

- Overall, levonorgestrel EHC prevents 85% of expected pregnancies if used within 72 hours of unprotected intercourse, but effectiveness declines with time. It is:
- 95% effective if the first dose is taken within 24 hours
- 85% effective if used within 24–48 hours
- 58% effective if used within 48–72 hours.
- It is not licensed for use more than 72 hours after unprotected intercourse.

Dosage

- The tablet is taken as soon as possible after unprotected sexual intercourse, preferably within 12 hours and not more than 72 hours after.
- Unprotected intercourse may have occurred because part of a course of an

oral contraceptive has been missed. In this situation, EHC can be offered if intercourse has taken place within 7 days of the following:
- with a combined contraceptive:
  - two or more pills missed from the first seven pills in a pack
  - four or more pills missed mid-course.

  If two or more pills are missed from the last seven in a pack, EHC is not necessary providing that the next pack is started immediately, i.e. without the normal pill-free break.
- with a progestogen-only contraceptive:
  - if one or more pills has been missed or taken more than 3 hours after the usual time.

- In all missed-pill situations, additional contraceptive precautions should be taken until consecutive daily pill-taking at the correct time has been resumed for at least 7 days.
- Taking levonorgestrel EHC may delay or bring forward the onset of the next period by a few days, but should not otherwise disrupt the cycle.
- Repeated courses are not dangerous, but can disrupt the cycle.
- Levonorgestrel EHC is not suitable as a regular means of contraception, and women who repeatedly ask for supplies should be advised to consider long-term methods.

Contraindications

There are very few situations in which levonorgestrel EHC cannot be safely recommended. The only contraindications are:
- hypersensitivity to levonorgestrel
- pregnancy, because it will be ineffective, although there is no evidence that the fetus will be harmed
- severe hepatic dysfunction
- conditions such as severe diarrhoea or Crohn's disease, where there is a high risk that the medication will not be absorbed.

A relative contraindication is breast cancer, although the risk to a sufferer from the medication is much less than that of pregnancy.

Breastfeeding is not a contraindication as only very small amounts of levonorgestrel appear in breast milk. (Any potential problem can be overcome by taking a dose immediately after feeding and not feeding the baby for at least 3 hours after taking a dose.)

Side-effects

- Side-effects of levonorgestrel EHC are as for progestogens generally and include abdominal pain, headache, dizziness, fatigue and breast tenderness, but these are not usually serious.
- The main undesirable effect is nausea, which affects about one-quarter of subjects, with vomiting occurring in about 5%. If vomiting occurs within 3 hours of a dose, absorption is impaired and another dose must be taken as soon as possible. A dose must be kept down for at least 3 hours within 84 hours of intercourse to ensure effectiveness.

Interactions

- Levonorgestrel is metabolised in the liver and drugs, including primidone, phenytoin, carbamazepine, St John's wort, griseofulvin, rifampicin, rifabutin and ritonavir, that induce liver enzymes will increase its metabolism and may reduce its effectiveness.
- Levonorgestrel inhibits the metabolism of ciclosporin, raising plasma levels and increasing the risk of toxicity.
- Patients taking any of these drugs should be referred to their doctor.

Self-assessment

Case study

An irate woman confronts you in the pharmacy. She brandishes an empty packet of the 'morning-after pill' at you and says she found it when she was cleaning her 15-year-old daughter's bedroom, and it has been dispensed at your pharmacy. She says that the general practitioner who prescribed it had no right to do so and you had no right to dispense it without asking her permission, as her daughter is still a child and is her responsibility and under her parental control. She says she is going to report both you and the general practitioner to 'the authorities'. What is your response?

Multiple choice questions

1. (Closed-book, simple completion)
    Which one of the following statements about EHC is incorrect?
    a. Overall, it prevents about 85% of expected pregnancies if used within 72 hours of unprotected intercourse.
    b. It is about 95% effective if the first dose is taken within 24 hours.
    c. It is about 85% effective if used within 24–48 hours.
    d. It is about 60% effective if used within 48–72 hours.
    e. The tablet should be taken 12 hours after unprotected intercourse.

2. (Closed-book, multiple completion)
    A woman wants to buy EHC because she has missed taking her combined oral contraceptive tablets. You should recommend it if intercourse has taken place within 7 days of the following:
    a   two or more pills missed from the first seven pills in a pack
    b. four or more pills missed mid-course
    c. two or more pills missed from the last seven in a pack

3. (Closed-book, assertion/reason)
    First statement: In all missed-pill situations, additional contraceptive precautions should be taken until consecutive daily pill-taking at the correct time has been resumed for at least 7 days.
    Second statement: Ovulation usually occurs around day 14 of a 28-day menstrual cycle.

Tips

In the registration exam calculators are not allowed. Calculation questions are designed to make sure that answers can be worked out fairly easily without a calculator, but you do have to be able to manipulate the basic arithmetic functions (addition, subtraction, multiplication and division). The best way to ensure this is to practise, practise, practise.

Definitions

- Premenstrual syndrome: distressing physical, psychological and behavioural symptoms not caused by organic disease, that regularly recur during the same phase of the menstrual cycle and significantly regress or disappear during the remainder of the cycle.
- The term 'premenstrual dysphoric disorder' (PMDD) describes a condition with more severe symptoms, which can cause major disruption to life and relationships.

Causes

- The cause of PMS (also known as premenstrual tension, PMT) is unknown, but it is associated with ovulation as it does not occur before puberty, during pregnancy or after the menopause, or in women who do not ovulate.
- One theory is that women with PMS are abnormally sensitive to progesterone secreted following ovulation, and that this reduces levels of pyridoxine. Pyridoxine is a coenzyme in the final step of the biosynthesis of serotonin, a neurotransmitter known to have potent effects on mood, and its deficiency may contribute to the depressive symptoms.

Epidemiology

- It is estimated that about 80% of menstruating women suffer some adverse symptoms prior to menstruation. Forty per cent of women have PMS, 10% severely enough to require treatment.
- Patients are usually over 30 years of age and symptoms often worsen with age until the menopause.
- The condition may become evident following childbirth or a disturbing life event.
- PMDD is believed to affect around 3–5% of women of reproductive age.

Signs and symptoms

Physical

- fluid retention and weight gain
- breast tenderness and fullness
- bloated abdomen
- change in bowel habit.

Psychological

- irritability
- anxiety
- depression
- changes in sleep, appetite and libido
- tiredness.

Behavioural

Women may be more prone to accidents, suicides and criminal activity.

Differential diagnosis

PMDD is diagnosed if at least five of the above signs and symptoms have been present to a marked degree in the week before menstruation for most months of the previous year.

Symptoms and circumstances for referral

Refer if 3 months of over-the-counter treatment have been ineffective.

Treatment

Prescription treatments

- Combined oral contraceptives prevent ovulation and are sometimes effective in treating PMS.
- Progestogens alone are also used, although clinical evidence has shown them to be of only marginal benefit.
- Serotonin transporter blockers have improved symptoms in some cases, particularly in women with underlying depressive illness.
- Non-steroidal anti-inflammatory drugs: naproxen and mefenamic acid taken during the luteal phase of the menstrual cycle have been found effective in some cases.

Non-prescription treatments

Pyridoxine

- Doses of pyridoxine of up to 100 mg/day are likely to be of benefit in treating premenstrual symptoms and premenstrual depression.

- The recommended dose is 100–200 mg daily for 3 days before the onset of symptoms until 2 days after the start of menstruation, or 50–100 mg daily throughout the month.
- Patients should be warned to be aware of signs of toxicity, such as tingling or numbness in the hands and feet, as very high doses can lead to peripheral neuropathies.
- Treatment should be discontinued if no benefit is perceived within 3 months.

Ammonium chloride
- A proprietary product is available containing ammonium chloride and caffeine, as a mild diuretic for premenstrual water retention.
- Reducing sodium and water intake for a few days before a period may reduce fluid retention as effectively.

Agnus castus (chaste tree) fruit extract
- Agnus castus has traditionally been used to relieve the symptoms of PMS and other menstrual problems, and compounds similar in structure to the sex hormones have been isolated from some parts of the plant.
- A clinical trial found agnus castus to be effective across a range of premenstrual symptoms.
- No preparations of agnus castus are available as licensed medicines, but there are products marketed as food supplements.

Self-assessment

Case study

A regular customer of yours, a woman in her 30s, comes into your pharmacy crying and distraught and asking for your help. Once you have calmed her a little and taken her to the private consultation area, she explains that she has been suffering from PMT for nearly 2 years, and it seems to be getting worse. Last night she was so bad that she physically attacked her husband for no reason. You ask if she has seen her general practitioner; she answers yes, but that nothing he prescribed has helped. She asks you if you know of anything that might help her. On checking her patient medical record you discover that her general practitioner has tried her successively on an oral contraceptive, dydrogesterone and amitriptyline during the past year. Is there anything that you could suggest?

Multiple choice questions
1–3.(Closed-book, classification)
   Questions 1–3 concern medical terminology:
a. amenorrhoea
b. dysmenorrhoea
c. menorrhagia
d. menorrhoea
e. menses

Which of the above terms describes:

1. normal menstrual flow?
2. abnormal absence of menstrual flow?
3. abnormally excessive menstrual flow?

4. (Open-book, multiple completion)
   Which of the drugs below is indicated for the treatment of premenstrual syndrome?
a. dydrogesterone
b. pyridoxine
c. tibolone

Tips

For the registration examination, get to know the *British National Formulary*, *Medicines Ethics and Practice* and *Drug Tariff* like the back of your hand! Thoroughly knowing your way around these reference sources will save you valuable time in the open-book paper.

chapter 34
Vaginal thrush

Causes

- Vaginal thrush (vulvovaginal candidiasis) is caused by a yeast, *Candida albicans*, a usually harmless inhabitant of the gastrointestinal tract, skin and vagina, which overgrows to cause infections when conditions allow.
- The vagina harbours an extensive flora of bacteria and fungi. In women of child-bearing age, oestrogen promotes the production of glycogen in the vaginal epithelium. The glycogen breaks down to glucose and lowers the pH of vaginal secretions, promoting an environment favourable to the growth of *Candida*.
- Predisposing factors for susceptibility to attacks include:
- pregnancy
- diabetes
- broad-spectrum antibiotics
- immunocompromised status
- immunosuppressant drugs, including oral steroids
- use of bath additives, vaginal deodorants and preparations for vulval pruritus containing local anaesthetics
- wearing occlusive underwear.

Epidemiology

Three-quarters of women suffer an episode at least once in their life, and 40–50% have more than one episode.

Signs and symptoms

- irritation or itching in the vulvovaginal area, often intense and burning. The external skin may be excoriated and raw from scratching
- vaginal discharge, either creamy-coloured, thick and curdy in appearance or thin and rather watery, but with no offensive odour
- there may be stinging on passing water due to inflammation of the vulva but otherwise no pain, and there is no increased frequency or urgency of micturition
- the vulva may be reddened and swollen.

Differential diagnosis

Conditions with symptoms that may be confused with vulvovaginal candidiasis include:

- Bacterial vaginosis: vaginitis (vaginal inflammation) caused by a combination of bacterial species usually present at low counts in the vagina, which when present at higher levels disrupt the normal flora and cause infection. Discharge may be confused with thrush, but it is white and watery with a strong 'fishy' odour. Itching is a less prominent feature than in candidiasis.
- Trichomoniasis: a sexually transmitted disease caused by a protozoan parasite, *Trichomonas vaginalis*. As in thrush, there is vulvar itching, but discharge is profuse, frothy, yellow-green in colour and with an unpleasant odour.
- Cystitis: with thrush, discomfort when urinating may be confused with dysuria associated with cystitis. However, in thrush the discomfort and burning are in the external vaginal area rather than in the bladder and urethra, as in cystitis.
- Atrophic vaginitis: in postmenopausal women lack of oestrogen reduces vaginal resistance to infection and injury, which can produce similar burning and itching symptoms to thrush, but thrush is uncommon in postmenopausal women.
- Adverse drug reactions: drugs that can predispose to thrush include broad-spectrum antibiotics, corticosteroids and drugs that can affect oestrogen levels, including oral contraceptives, hormone replacement therapy, tamoxifen and raloxifene.

Symptoms and circumstances for referral

- If vaginal candidiasis has not been previously diagnosed by a doctor. There are other vaginal infections, some serious and all requiring treatment with prescription-only medication, with symptoms that could be confused with thrush. An initial medical diagnosis of candidiasis is necessary so that sufferers can recognise the condition subsequently.
- Patients with recurrent attacks: more than two within the previous 6 months may indicate an underlying cause such as diabetes.
- Patients under 16 or over 60 years of age: thrush is rare in these age groups due to the lack of vaginal oestrogen, which favours growth of *C. albicans*, but lack of oestrogen increases susceptibility to other vaginal infections. Over-the-counter (OTC) treatments are not licensed for use in these groups.
- Pregnant or breastfeeding women: OTC treatments are not licensed for use in these groups.
- Abnormal or irregular vaginal bleeding.
- Any blood staining of vaginal discharge.
- Vulval or vaginal sores, ulcers or blisters.
- Lower abdominal pain or dysuria, which may indicate a urinary tract infection.
- Patients with a previous history of sexually transmitted disease or exposure to a partner with such a history, as other infections may be present.
- No improvement after treatment with OTC medication.
- All the above are criteria for referral to a doctor and form part of the licensing conditions for non-prescription sale of azole anticandidal treatments.

Treatment

Most treatments for vaginal thrush are available without prescription.

Azoles

- Azoles are synthetic antimycotic agents that act by inhibiting replication of yeast cells through interfering with the synthesis of ergosterol, the main sterol in the yeast cell membrane.
- Azoles available without prescription for treatment of vaginal thrush are fluconazole, clotrimazole and econazole.

Fluconazole

- Fluconazole is presented as a single-dose 150 mg oral capsule.
- It is well absorbed when taken by mouth, and symptoms usually improve 12–24 hours after administration.
- Adverse effects are generally mild and mainly gastrointestinal, including abdominal pain, diarrhoea, nausea and vomiting and flatulence.
- Fluconazole interacts with a number of drugs, including those metabolised by cytochrome P450 enzymes, but interactions are unlikely to be clinically significant with a single dose of fluconazole.

Clotrimazole

- Clotrimazole is only used topically because of adverse effects when given orally and varying absorption rates, and because it is metabolised in the liver to inactive compounds.
- It is available for intravaginal use as a single 500 mg pessary, a 5 g prefilled single application of 10% cream, and 2% cream available for twice or three times daily application to the external genitalia.
- Symptoms usually begin to improve more quickly than with oral fluconazole.
- The bases used in some preparations damage latex condoms and diaphragms.
- Night-time use is recommended for intravaginal preparations as the patient will be lying down for several hours, allowing the drug a chance to act and avoiding the problems of seepage and loss that would occur if the patient was upright and moving around.

Econazole

Econazole is licensed for non-prescription sale only for topical external use, and is available as a 1% cream.

Povidone-iodine

- Povidone-iodine is an iodophore in which povidone, a vinyl polymer, acts as a carrier for iodine, allowing its gradual release for antimicrobial and antiseptic effect. It is less potent than preparations containing free iodine but is less toxic.
- Povidone-iodine has activity against a wide range of microorganisms, including fungi, but is less effective than the azoles and requires twice-daily administration for up to 14 days.
- It is available as 200 mg pessaries and a 10% solution, which should be diluted 1:10 with water before use as an intravaginal wash.

Additional advice

- Sexual intercourse should be avoided until cure is complete, to avoid transfer of infection and reinfection.
- Candida infection can be transferred from the bowel; after bowel movements the anus should be wiped from front to back to help prevent transfer of organisms.
- Women susceptible to attacks should:
- keep the vulva cool and dry by careful hygiene, use of cotton rather than synthetic underwear and careful drying after washing the vaginal area, as the infection thrives in a moist, warm environment
- avoid use of foam baths, douches and vaginal deodorants, which can strip away the protective lining of the vagina.

Self-assessment

Case study

You are called by your medicines counter assistant to talk to a young woman who wants to buy a fluconazole capsule but has not had it before. When you ask her why she wants it she says that she thinks she has thrush. When you ask her how she knows, she says because her friend has told her that's what it must be. When you ask her to describe her symptoms more fully, she tells you that for the past 2 days she has had intense itching inside and outside her vagina. She also has a thick, creamy discharge, but there is no unpleasant odour. She experiences some burning on the outside when she passes water, but otherwise feels well with no fever or other symptoms, but she has just got over a nasty throat infection and about a week ago had a prescription for amoxicillin dispensed at your pharmacy. Will you sell her the fluconazole?

Multiple choice questions

1. (Closed-book, multiple completion)

   Assuming that there were no other factors preventing supply, to which of the following could a fluconazole 150 mg capsule for the treatment of vaginal thrush not be sold?

   a. a girl aged 16 years
   b. a woman aged 57 years
   c. a woman aged 62 years

2. (Open-book, assertion/reason)

   First statement: For systemic treatment of vaginal candidiasis in a patient with liver disease, itraconazole is preferable to fluconazole.
   Second statement: Itraconazole is less hepatotoxic than fluconazole.

Tips

Maximise your chances in an exam by eliminating avoidable pressure-causing factors that can lead to a poor performance. Try to get a good night's sleep the night before, don't revise into the early hours and plan to arrive early to allow time for possible travel delays.

Answers to self-assessment

2 Cardiovascular conditions
Case study

From the information this man gives, he is not within the groups for whom simvastatin is licensed for over-the-counter sale and he could just be given reassurance or referred to his general practitioner if he is still worried. On the other hand, you may consider that there is little or no risk in his taking simvastatin and that he could be sold the product for his peace of mind. However, in doing this you would be supplying the product outside its licensing conditions and would be taking personal responsibility for its supply.

Multiple choice questions
1. c (*BNF*, Appendix 1)
2. b (*MEP*, List of medicines for human use, table: Aspirin legal status)
3. a (*MEP*, List of medicines for human use, table: Aspirin legal status)

3 Motion sickness
Case study

Cinnarizine is a suitable choice. Hyoscine has more pronounced antimuscarinic side-effects and requires 4-hourly dosing. Drowsiness and antimuscarinic side-effects with cinnarizine are not usually a problem; it requires 8-hourly dosing and it will not interact with the patient's medication. Evidence of effectiveness of ginger is conflicting and it may be best not to try it for the first time on a very long journey.

Multiple choice questions
1. a (*BNF*)
2. b (*BNF*)

4 Pain
1. c
2. d
3. b
4. c (*MEP*)

5 Ear problems
Case study

The patient suffers barotrauma, caused by pressure on the eardrum as the air pressure in the cabin increases on the aircraft's descent. It is more likely to be suffered by people who have had repeated ear infections in childhood, or who have suffered inner-ear damage or injury from other causes. It is also worsened by a current or recent upper respiratory tract infection. It is often relieved by use of a decongestant nasal spray just before descent begins or an oral decongestant (e.g. pseudoephedrine) taken about an hour before descent. Chewing or sucking (e.g. a toffee or boiled sweet) or yawning also helps to equalise pressure in the eustachian tube and ease pain. Valsalva's manoeuvre can also be used: the nostrils are held tightly closed with the thumb and forefinger while the person tries to blow out through the nose with the mouth closed.

Multiple choice questions

1. d (*BNF*)
2. b
3. b (*BNF, Drug Tariff* part XVIIIA)
4. a (*BNF*)
5. b (*BNF*)

6 Eye conditions
Case study

The patient probably has a chalazion (meibomian cyst), which can develop following a stye. It may enlarge and grow inwards and start to rub against the eye surface. Removal is usually a simple process under local anaesthetic. There is no treatment you can suggest but you can advise him to see his doctor to arrange to have it removed.

Multiple choice questions

1. d
2. d (*BNF*)
3. e (*BNF*)
4. d (*BNF*)
5. b

7 Athlete's foot
Case study

- A terbinafine preparation may be the most suitable – although an imidazole would probably be as effective, the length of treatment with terbinafine is shorter.
- Whichever treatment you recommend, emphasise the need to use it for the full period of treatment advised by the manufacturer. Infections often return because patients stop treatment as soon as symptoms subside and before the infection has been completely eradicated.
- Advise on foot hygiene measures:
- Wash and thoroughly dry feet and toes daily, particularly between the toes.
- Do not share towels in communal changing rooms.
- Wash towels frequently.
- Change socks daily.

- Wear flip-flops or plastic sandals in communal changing rooms and showers.
- When at home leave shoes and socks off as much as possible.
- Avoid occlusive footwear such as trainers, if possible.
- Use an antifungal powder or spray inside socks and shoes each time before putting them on.

Multiple choice questions

1. d (answer self-explanatory from text)
2. c (*BNF*)
3. c (*BNF*)
4. a (*BNF*)

8 Foot (podiatric) problems
Case study

Tell the young woman that her grandmother should not try to treat herself and that she should see a chiropodist. (Reasons are given in the chapter.)

Multiple choice questions

1. c (*BNF* and *Drug Tariff*. Duofilm is licensed for mosaic and plantar warts only; corn rings are listed as a chiropody appliance in *Drug Tariff* part IXA, and are prescribable)
2. e (*BNF*, section 13.7)

9 Fungal nail infection (onychomycosis)
Case study

The 'new' product is amoralfine 5% nail lacquer, which was reclassified from prescription-only medicine (POM) to P in May 2006. You could advise the customer that her general practitioner could prescribe it for her on the NHS and she would not have to pay for it.

Multiple choice questions

1. d (*BNF*, *Drug Tariff*). Curanail is prescribable on the NHS: although it is not listed in the *BNF*, neither is it listed in part XVIIIA of the *Drug Tariff* (the 'black list').

10 Verrucas (plantar warts) and warts (common warts)
Case study

Firstly, you should check that she has been using the salicylic acid preparations properly and for long enough. Even if she has been using them properly, it would take up to about 3 months to get rid of the verruca. Her other options now are to do nothing, and the chances are that the verruca will go of its own accord within the next few months or have the verruca removed with cryotherapy, which should work immediately, although the area is likely to be quite sore for several days after treatment.

Multiple choice questions

1. d (*BNF*)
2. b (*BNF*)
3. d (*BNF*)
4. a (*BNF*)

11 Constipation
Case study

The patient's constipation could be caused by dihydrocodeine in the co-dydramol tablets; constipation is a common side-effect of opiate analgesics. You could suggest that she try taking paracetamol alone, to see if that cured the constipation. If it did but did not control the arthritic pain sufficiently, you could suggest that she stays on co-dydramol and asks her general practitioner to prescribe a laxative – lactulose may be appropriate – for the constipation.

Multiple choice questions

1. e (*BNF*)
2. b (*BNF*)
3. a (*BNF*)
4. a (both statements are true and a is a consequence of b)

12 Diarrhoea
Case study

The boy probably has acute diarrhoea. No treatment should be needed, but the mother should be advised to make sure that her son is drinking plenty of fluids. If the diarrhoea has not stopped or is not lessening after another 24 hours, she should take her son to the doctor.

Multiple choice questions

1. a (*BNF*)
2. d (*BNF*)
3. e (*BNF*)
4. d

13 Haemorrhoids (piles)
Case study

The woman's symptoms strongly suggest haemorrhoids, and you should strongly recommend her to see her doctor to have your diagnosis confirmed. If she is still unwilling to do so, you could advise her to continue with her high-fibre diet but to make sure that she has plenty of fluids as well, as fibre without fluid may form a dry mass in the intestine that can contribute to constipation and haemorrhoids. You could also recommend a soothing and astringent haemorrhoid cream or ointment, with the advice that if the condition does not improve within a week she must see her doctor.

Multiple choice questions
1. b (Anusol-HC ointment is a prescription-only medicine, but Anusol Plus HC ointment is the same and can be sold without prescription: *BNF*)
2. c

14 Irritable-bowel syndrome (IBS)
Case study
The woman should be referred to her general practitioner, as her symptoms are causing general debilitation and should be investigated again. A possibility that is sometimes overlooked initially is a malabsorption condition such as coeliac disease.

Multiple choice questions
1. b
2. a

15 Indigestion
Case study
The patient would need to be referred to her doctor for her medication to be reviewed as the indigestion may be the result of gastric irritation as a side-effect of the diclofenac. You could recommend to the doctor that, as the diclofenac appears to be working well, and providing there are no other adverse factors, he could continue to prescribe it together with a proton pump inhibitor to protect against gastric ulceration.

Multiple choice questions
1. d (Tolterodine is an antimuscarinic used in the management of urinary frequency and urgency; zidovudine is a nucleoside reverse transcriptase inhibitor used in the management of human immunodeficiency virus (HIV) infection)
2. e (*BNF*)
3. c (2 could indicate a peptic ulcer and 3 myocardial ischaemia)

16 Mouth ulcers (minor aphthous ulcers)
Case study
No. This person should be referred to a doctor immediately, as there are several referral factors in the history and symptoms he describes and the appearance of the lesion. They may indicate a squamous cell carcinoma.

Multiple choice questions
1. a
2. a (*BNF*. The 10 g pack of Adcortyl in Orabase is prescription-only medicine, the 5 g pack is P)

17 Head lice
Case study

You should inform the woman that using malathion shampoo is unlikely to prevent the family catching head lice. Instead, she should check family members' heads twice weekly by wet combing (explaining to her how to do it if she does not know) until the outbreak is over, and if she detects anyone with signs of infestation to treat them with a pediculicide. But she should only treat those who are infested, not the rest of the family. Advise her against using malathion shampoo for eradication as it is much less effective than other preparations.

Multiple choice questions

1. a
2. c (*BNF*)
3. d (*BNF*)
4. a (*BNF*)
5. a (*BNF*)

18 Scabies
Case study

There is no doubt that the children are at risk, although not everyone who is in contact with scabies gets it. You should advise the woman to treat her children prophylactically now, as if they have been infected it could be some weeks before they have any symptoms. There is no need to go to her general practitioner as you can sell her a scabicide without prescription, unless she wants to save money and go to the doctor for a prescription.

Multiple choice questions

1. b (*BNF*)
2. c (*BNF*)
3. d (*BNF*)

19 Threadworm
Case study

It is most likely that the child is reinfecting himself. You could remind her to make sure that she is doing the following:

- putting on underpants under his pyjamas, so that he is less likely to pick up eggs on his fingers at night through scratching the anal area
- giving him a bath in the morning to wash away any eggs that may have been laid overnight
- keeping his fingernails trimmed short and making sure he washes his hands and scrubs his fingers with a nailbrush every time he goes to the toilet and before he eats, so that he does not ingest any eggs he may be carrying
- giving him a second dose of anthelmintic medication a fortnight after the first to kill off any worms that may not have been killed by the first dose
- treating all the family with anthelmintic medication to make sure that they do not become infected and continue the cycle of infection.

Multiple choice questions
1. a

20 Musculoskeletal conditions
Case study
1. The woman appears to be suffering from muscle strain. You could recommend an over-the-counter analgesic: ibuprofen might be the most effective, so long as she is not hypersensitive to it. She should also take a few days off work to allow her muscles to recover, and heat treatment such as hot baths may help.
2. This man may have broken his ankle. You should advise him to go to the Accident & Emergency department.

Multiple choice questions
1. c

21 Common cold and influenza
Case study
The symptoms are indicative of influenza and he may have developed a secondary bacterial chest infection. He is also considered an at-risk patient because of his age and his cardiovascular conditions. For these reasons you should tell his daughter to contact his doctor immediately.

Multiple choice questions
1. d (*BNF*)
2. c
3. c (*BNF*)
4. c (*BNF*)

22 Cough
Case study
It is not uncommon for coughs to persist for several weeks in children after a chest infection. However, the child may have an allergy and be developing asthma. If so, the most likely cause is house dust mite or dander (fur particles) from a household pet. You should ask the mother for further clues; for example: is he worse in any particular room of the house, or worse after dust is raised, say with vacuuming or with changing the bed sheets? Do any other family members suffer from asthma, hayfever or eczema? On the other hand the child may have another viral upper respiratory tract infection, but as you are unable to decide the cause you should advise the mother to take him back to the doctor.

Multiple choice questions
1. c (a, b and d are not prescribable on the NHS, e is not indicated for non-productive cough. *Drug Tariff*, part XVIIIA; *BNF*)
2. c
3. b
4. e

23 Hayfever
Case study

Sodium cromoglicate eye drops and nasal spray may be helpful, as cumulative experience suggests that it has no effect on fetal development. However, as the patient is already under medical supervision, she should be referred back to her general practitioner or obstetrician to prescribe them. To help with the nasal congestion, you could suggest that the patient tries steam inhalations, using menthol or other suitable inhalants.

Multiple choice questions

1. d (*BNF*)
2. c (*BNF*)
3. a (*BNF*)
4. e (cetirizine is the only non-sedating histamine, all the others are sedating)

24 Nicotine replacement therapy (NRT)
Case study

You should tell him that Zyban (bupropion hydrochloride) is a prescription-only medicine and he would need a prescription from his doctor for it. Zyban appears to be more effective than NRT but his doctor would need to assess whether it is suitable and safe for him to take, especially with the condition he is currently being treated for, as it is contraindicated in patients with central nervous system disorders and some mental conditions. Tell him also that offering Zyban for sale from a website in the UK would be in contravention of the Medicines Act and illegal, although most advertising comes from sites abroad. The customer should be strongly advised against buying Zyban from an e-mail offer, because it is quite likely to be a counterfeit, placebo or substitute drug.

Multiple choice questions

1. a
2. a (*Drug Tariff*; only Nicobrevin is listed in Part XVIIIA)
3. b
4. c
5. a

25 Acne
Case study

Hormonal contraceptives can be used to control acne. Co-cyprindiol, containing cyproterone, an antiandrogen that decreases sebum production, and ethinylestradiol is specifically indicated for women with moderate to severe acne, but it is not available without prescription.

Multiple choice questions

1. a (*BNF*. Differin is the only preparation in the list that is denoted prescription-ony medicine)
2. b (*Drug Tariff*, part XVIIIA ('the blacklist'))

3.   e (no improvement after 2 months with over-the-counter treatment is a factor for referral, but the other two factors are not necessarily)

26 Cold sores (oral herpes simplex)
Case study
- Put the woman's mind at rest by telling her that almost anyone who has touched or kissed the child could have passed on the virus to her, and that it is virtually impossible to avoid being infected as about 80% of people carry the virus.
- As cold and wind seemed to be a trigger for her daughter's only attack, she should take precautions to protect the child's face and mouth in such conditions. She should also not let her daughter's skin dry out in cold weather, as infection can begin in cracked skin.
- To prevent her son getting an infection from his sister, she should make sure that he does not share her cup or cutlery when she has active cold sores, but it is not necessary at other times: although the virus is still present, it is inactive.

Multiple choice questions
1.   d (*BNF*)
2.   e (*BNF*)
3.   c (*MEP*, Alphabetical List of Medicines for Human Use)

27 Eczema/dermatitis
Case study
The rash would appear to be due to a mild exacerbation of atopic eczema. You could recommend an emollient cream with advice that if the rash has not improved in another few days, the mother should take the child to their doctor.

Multiple choice questions
1.   c
2.   a
3.   e
4.   c

28 Fungal skin infections
Case study
The symptoms could describe pityriasis versicolor. Another possibility is vitiligo, but that is usually more widespread and also affects the face, there is no scaling and the skin does not itch. You could recommend an imidazole cream, e.g. clotrimazole, applied daily for 3 weeks. If the condition has not improved by then, he should go back to his doctor and ask to be referred to a dermatologist.

Multiple choice questions
1.   b
2.   c
3.   d
4.   c (*BNF*. Nizoral cream should not be dispensed unless the prescription is endorsed Selected List Scheme (SLS) by the prescriber)

29 Scalp conditions
Case study

The man may have seborrhoeic dermatitis, for which there is no cure, although treatment is usually able to control the more troublesome features. If he has tried several over-the-counter treatments without success, he may find that shampooing his hair daily with an ordinary mild shampoo will control the situation just as well as, or better than, anything else. If this does not work either, he should be referred to his general practitioner.

Multiple choice questions

1. e (from text: *Pediculus humanus capitis* infection is head lice)
2. e
3. c
4. c

30 Cystitis
Case study

The symptoms are not typical of cystitis and may indicate a kidney infection. No medicine should be sold and the patient should immediately be referred to a doctor.

Multiple choice questions

1. c
2. b (BNF)
3. c (first statement is true; second statement: potassium salts do not cause fluid retention and raise blood pressure, so it is false)

31 Dysmenorrhoea
Case study

The symptoms described indicate primary dysmenorrhoea, so you could recommend treatment. Ibuprofen is the best analgesic to recommend, but check first that the girl is not sensitive to it. If ibuprofen is not effective after trying it for a couple of months she should see her doctor.

Multiple choice questions

1. b (BNF)
2. e (information in text)
3. c (information in text. Non-steroidal anti-inflammatory drugs act by blocking the enzyme cyclo-oxygenase)

32 Emergency hormonal contraception
Case study

The law relating to confidentiality and consent in this kind of situation has been tested in the courts, and it has been established that girls under 16 (the legal age for consent to sexual intercourse) can be considered competent to seek medical advice and to consent to treatment without parental knowledge or consent. The Data Protection Act and the Royal Pharmaceutical Society's Code of Ethics prohibit disclosure of confidential information about a 'competent' person to a third party without the person's consent. You should tactfully explain the situation to the mother.

Multiple choice questions

1. e
2. b
3. b

33 Premenstrual syndrome (PMS)
Case study

There is evidence of effectiveness for pyridoxine, which is available without prescription, and is worth a try (see text for dosage) for 3 months. If that fails, agnus castus extract might be worth trying.

Multiple choice questions

1. d
2. a
3. c
4. b (*BNF*)

34 Vaginal thrush
Case study

The young woman has described classic symptoms of an attack of thrush that appears to have been triggered by the recent use of a broad-spectrum antibiotic. But you cannot supply the fluconazole as the licensing conditions prohibit over-the-counter sale unless the condition has been previously diagnosed by a doctor, which has not been the case for this patient.

Multiple choice questions

1. e (over-the-counter treatments for vaginal thrush may not be sold without prescription for patients under the age of 16 or over 60 years)
2. e (*BNF*, section 5.2)

Glossary

angioedema	an allergic or hypersensitivity reaction, manifesting as circumscribed patches of swelling on the skin and mucous membranes
atheromatous	from atheroma, an abnormal fatty deposit in an artery
atherosclerosis	blocking and hardening of the coronary arteries caused by the presence of atheromas
atopy	susceptibility to allergic-type reaction without external cause. Examples of atopic conditions are asthma and eczema
bilateral	on both sides
cariogenic	causing dental decay
conjunctiva	the mucous membrane lining the inner surface of the eyelid and the front of the eyeball
cornea	the transparent part of the coat of the eyeball, covering the iris and pupil
dermis	the sensitive vascular inner layer of the skin
dyscrasia	usually refers to an abnormality in a component of the blood
dysphagia	difficulty in swallowing
dyspnoea	difficulty in breathing; shortness of breath
dystrophy	abnormal or defective growth
embolism	the sudden obstruction of a blood vessel by an air bubble or other abnormal particle
encephalopathy	disease of the brain
endogenous	caused by factors within the body
epigastric	the area around the stomach
erythema	abnormal redness of the skin
excoriation	destruction of areas of skin surface, e.g. by scratching
fontanelle	in babies, areas of the head in which bone has not yet formed. The main one of these is the anterior fontanelle situated at the top of the skull. It normally closes by the age of 18 months
frontal	across the forehead
hypertrophy	excessive growth
hyphae (plural of hypha)	long, slender branched filaments that are an element of fungal structure
ischaemic	from ischaemia, describing the absence of arterial blood supply to a part of the body
maceration	the softening of tissue by the action of moisture
myalgia	muscle pains

mycelial	from mycelium, the structure formed from the mass of interwoven fungal hyphae (see hyphae)
myelosuppression	suppression of the bone marrow's production of blood cells and platelets
myocardium	the muscular layer of the heart wall
neuropathy	an abnormal and usually degenerative state of the nervous system or nerves
occipital	at the base of the skull
ocular	around the eyes
papule	a small solid elevation of the skin caused by inflammation, accumulated secretion or hypertrophy (excessive growth) of tissue
paroxysm	an attack of sudden onset
pinna	the largely cartilaginous projecting portion of the external ear
pleurisy	inflammation of the pleura, the membrane forming the outer lining of the lungs
prodrome	warning signs, usually occurring within an hour or two of the start of a migraine attack. May be visual (blind spots, flashes, zig-zag lines), neurological (pins and needles or numbness in the hand, arm or face), yawning or food cravings
prolapse	the falling or slipping down of a body part from its usual position
pustule	a small circumscribed elevation of the skin containing pus and having an inflamed base
sacral	relating to the sacrum, the vertebra at the lower end of the spine connecting it to the pelvis
thrombosis	a blood clot within a blood vessel
tinnitus	a sensation of noise, e.g. ringing, buzzing in the ear
unilateral	on one side
URTI	upper respiratory tract infection
vertigo	dizziness caused by several disorders, often of the inner ear
vitiligo	a skin disorder in which patches of skin lose their pigment and become white as a result of a reduction in the production of melanin

Index

acetic acid 2% spray solution, 34
aciclovir, 170-1
acne (acne vulgaris), 163-8
acrivastine, 150, 176
adsorbent antidiarrhoeal agents, 79
agnus castus (chaste tree) fruit extract, 209
air travel, 19, 33
alcohol consumption, 12, 19
alginates, 98
alkalinising agents, urinary, 194-5
allantoin, 85
allergic conjunctivitis, 37, 148
allergic contact dermatitis, 173, 174-5, 176
Aluminium Acetate 13% Ear Drops BP, 34
aluminium-containing antacids, 68, 96, 97, 98
alverine citrate, 90
amantidine, 132
ammonium chloride, 142, 209
amorolfine 5nail lacquer, 58-9
anal fissure, 84
anal fistula, 84
analgesics, 24-7, 28, 33, 124-5, 133, 199-200
angina pectoris, 8-9, 95
angiotensin-converting enzyme inhibitors, 95,
    132, 140, 195
antacids, 95-8
antazoline sulphate, 152
anthraquinones, 70
antidepressants, 68, 142, 158
antiflatulents, 98
antifungal agents, 48-50, 180, 181, 188, 213
antihistamines, 18-19, 133, 141, 142, 149-50,
    152, 175, 176, 200
  non-sedating, 150, 176
  sedating, 26, 141, 142, 149-50, 176
antimicrobials, 39, 135, 166, 195
antimotility agents, 78-9, 90
antispasmodics, 90, 98
antitussives, 141-2, 144
antiviral agents, 170-1
aphthous ulcers, 101-3
artificial tears (tear substitutes), 41
aspirin, 8, 13, 24-5, 26, 28, 133, 199
  hypersensitivity, 24, 55, 79, 124, 125, 166,
    199
asthma, 24, 132, 140, 141, 148, 174
astringents, 41, 85, 86, 171
athlete's foot, 47-51
atopic eczema, 173, 174, 186
atropine, 79, 98

attapulgite, 79
azoles, 213

back pain, 123, 125-6
bacterial conjunctivitis, 37, 39
bacterial vaginosis, 212
barotrauma, 33
basal cell carcinoma, 42, 62
beclometasone, 151
benzidamine, 102, 124
benzocaine, 84, 135
benzoic acid, 49-50
benzoyl peroxide, 165
benzyl benzoate, 114
beta-blockers, 133, 140, 143, 158
bisacodyl, 70
bismuth oxide, 85
bismuth salicylate, 79, 96, 97
bismuth subgallate, 85
blackheads (open comedones), 163, 164
blepharitis, 41
blood in stool, 83, 84
breastfeeding, 58, 158, 212
  drug precautions/contraindications, 19, 25,
    27, 40, 70, 85, 99, 124, 151, 204
brompheniramine, 142
bronchitis, 132, 140, 141
buclizine, 26
bulk-forming laxatives, 69
bunions, 55

caffeine, 26, 200, 209
calcium carbonate antacids, 96
calluses, 53, 54-5
candidiasis, 101, 134, 211-14
carbimazole, 134
carbomer 940, 41
cardiovascular disease, 7-14, 158
  drug precautions/contraindications, 19, 24,
    27, 133, 143, 158, 195
cardiovascular risk factors, 11, 12, 27
carminatives, 98
cerumen (ear wax), 33-4
cerumenolytics, 33, 34
cetrimide, 166
cetrizine, 150, 176
chalazion (meibomian cyst), 41
chest pain, 7-8, 9
chickenpox, 101, 170
chloramphenicol, 39-40

chlorhexidine, 103, 166
chlorphenamine, 149, 176
chlorpromazine, 68
choline salicylate, 33, 171
cinchocaine, 84
cinnarazine, 18
clobetasone butyrate, 176
clotrimazole, 48, 213
clozapine, 134
cluster headache, 22, 23
coal tar preparations, 184, 185, 187
co-codamol, 26, 200
co-codaprin, 26, 200
co-cyprindiol, 167
co-danthramer, 70
co-danthrusate, 70
codeine, 26, 68, 142, 200
co-dydramol, 26, 200
cold sores, 169-72
comedolytics, 165
comedones, 163, 164, 167
common cold, 131-7, 149
conjunctivitis, 37, 39, 148
constipation, 26, 67-74, 83, 84, 86, 89, 90
contact dermatitis, 58, 173, 174-5, 176, 194
co-phenotrope, 79
corneal conditions, 37-40
corns, 53-5
corticosteroids, topical, 102, 151, 175, 187
co-trimazole, 134
cough, 139-45
counterirritants (rubefacients), 125, 171
cradle cap, 183, 185, 186-7
Crohn's disease, 75, 89, 204
crotamiton, 114
croup, 140
cryotherapy, warts/verrucas, 63
cyclo-oxygenase inhibitors, 13, 24, 25, 199
cystitis, 193-6, 212

dacryocystitis, 37
dandruff (pityriasis capitis), 183-5
dantron, 70
decongestants, 133, 143-4, 150, 152
demulcents, 134-5, 144
dental pain, 28
dermatitis, 173-7, 194
  seborrhoeic, 183, 184, 185-6
dermatophytes, 47, 57, 179
dextromethorphan, 142, 144
diabetic patients, 48, 54, 57, 58, 75, 158, 211,
  212
  drug precautions/contraindications, 72, 133,
  143, 195
diarrhoea, 68, 75-81, 89, 90, 204
dibromopropamidine isetionate, 39, 40, 41
diclofenac, 124
dicycloverine, 98

dihydrocodeine, 26, 68, 200
dimethyl ether and propane (DMEP), 63
dimeticone, 108-9
diphenhydramine, 142, 149, 200
diphenoxylate, 79
diphenylmethane derivatives, 70
distal and lateral subungual onychomycosis,
  57, 58
docusate, 34, 70, 72
domperidone, 99
drug reactions
  acne, 164
  blood dyscrasias, 132, 134
  constipation, 26, 67, 68
  cough, 140, 141
  diarrhoea, 75
  glaucoma, 152
  indigestion, 95
dry eye, 39, 41
dysentery, 75
dysmenorrhoea, 197-201
dysuria, 193, 212

ear problems, 33-5
ear wax, 33-4
earache, 33
econazole, 48, 213
eczema, 34, 48, 113, 173-7, 179
elderly people, 9, 10, 54, 67, 68, 132
  drug precautions, 19, 24, 71, 90, 142
emergency aid
  angina pectoris, 9
  heart failure, 10
  myocardial infarction (heart attack), 8
  stroke, 11
emergency hormonal contraception, 203-6
emollients, 175-6
ephedrine, 133, 143
epidermabrasion, 54
epilepsy, 19, 27, 117
episcleritis, 38
erythrasma, 48, 180
expectorants, 142-3, 144
eye conditions, 37-43
eye strain-related headache, 21, 22
eyelid conditions, 40-1

faecal impaction, 68
faecal lubricants, 72-3
faecal softeners, 72
famotidine, 98, 99
felbinac, 124
fever, 133
fibroids (fibromyomas), 198
fish oils, 13, 14
fluconazole, 213
flurbiprofen, 134, 135
fluticasone, 151

foot (podiatric) problems, 53-6
formaldehyde, 63
fungal infection, 175, 179-82
  see also athlete's foot; onychomycosis

gasteroenteritis (acute infective diarrhoea), 75, 76, 77-8
gastro-oesophageal reflux, 93, 140
giardiasis, 75, 76, 89
glandular fever (infectious mononucleosis), 132, 134
glaucoma, 19, 21, 27, 38, 90, 142, 143, 152
gluteraldehyde, 63
glycerol, 34, 72, 134, 144
glyceryl trinitrate, 9
grapefruit juice, 12
griseofulvin, 49, 188
guaifensin, 142, 143, 144

H2-antagonists, 98-9
haemorrhoids, 67, 68, 83-7, 117
hamamelis (witch hazel), 41, 85
hayfever, 147-53, 174
head lice, 107-11
headache, 10, 21-6, 148
heart attack (myocardial infarction), 7-8, 9
heart failure, 9-10, 71, 132, 140
heartburn see gastro-oesophageal reflux
herpes simplex, 101, 169-72
hordeolum (stye), 40-1
hydrocolloid plasters, 54
hydrocortisone, 34, 85, 86, 102, 176
hydrogel plasters, 54
hyoscine, 18, 19, 90
hypromellose, 41

ibuprofen, 24-5, 26, 28, 124, 133, 195, 199, 200
imidazoles, 48, 180, 181
imipramine, 68
immunocompromised patients, 57, 58, 61, 211
immunosuppressants, 175
impetigo, 170
indigestion, 93-100
inflammatory bowel disease, 75, 84, 89, 90
influenza, 131-7
ingrown toenail, 56
ipecacuanha, 142
iritis (uveitis), 38
irritable bowel syndrome, 68, 75, 89-91, 95
irritant dermatitis, 173, 176
isometheptene mucate, 27
isotretinoin, 167
ispaghula husk, 69, 90
itraconazole, 58, 97

kaolin, 79
keratitis (corneal ulcer), 38
keratolytics, 165

ketoconazole, 48, 97, 181, 184, 185
ketoprofen, 124

lactic acid, 62
lactose intolerance, 72, 79
lactulose, 71-2
lauromacrogol 400, 85
laxatives, 67, 68-73, 75, 83, 90
levonorgestrel, 203-6
lichen planus, 58
lidocaine, 84, 135, 171
liquid paraffin, 72-3
lithium, 25, 98, 164, 195
liver disease, drug contraindications, 24, 27, 117, 204
local anaesthetic preparations, 84-5, 103, 135, 171
lodoxamide, 152
loperamide, 78
loratadine, 150, 176
low back pain, 123, 125

macrogols (polyethylene glycols), 72
magnesium antacids, 96, 97, 98
magnesium hydroxide, 71
magnesium sulphate, 71
magnesium–alumnium antacids, 96
malabsorption syndromes, 75, 89
malathion, 108, 109, 110, 114
mast cell stabilisers, 151, 152
mebendazole, 117
mebeverine hydrochloride, 90
meclozine, 18
mefenamic acid, 208
meibomian cyst (chalazion), 41
meningitis, 21, 22, 132
menthol, 90, 125, 134, 171
methylcellulose, 69
methysergide, 27
metronidazole, 95
miconazole, 48
migraine, 21-7
mittelschmerz, 198
moclobemide, 27
moisturisers, 175-6
monoamine oxidase inhibitors, 27, 133, 143
morphine, 68, 78-9
motion sickness, 17-20
mouth ulcers, 101-3, 170
musculoskeletal conditions, 123-7
myocardial infarction (heart attack), 7-8, 9, 13
myocarditis, 9

nail disorders, 56, 58
  see also onychomycosis
naphazoline eye drops, 41
naproxen, 208
nasal congestion, 133, 148, 150, 151, 152

nicotinamide, 166
nicotine replacement therapy, 155-9
nitrofurantoin, 97, 195
non-steroidal anti-inflammatory drugs
   (NSAIDs), 24-5, 95, 124, 140, 199, 208
Norwalk virus diarrhoea, 76

omega-3 triglycerides, 13-14
omeprazole, 99
onychomycosis, 47, 57-60
opioids, 26, 68, 141, 142, 200
oral contraceptives, 204, 208
oral rehydration therapy, 77-8, 80
oral thrush, 101, 134
orphenadrine, 68, 142
oseltamivir, 132
osmotic laxatives, 71-2
otitis externa, 34
otitis media, 33, 148
oxymetazoline, 133, 152

pain, 21-9
   on defaecation, 83, 84
   dental, 28
   irritable bowel syndrome, 89
   low back, 123, 125
paracetamol, 25, 26, 27, 28, 133, 195, 199, 200
paradichlorobenzene, 34
paronychia, 56
pelvic inflammatory disease, 198
penciclovir, 171
penicillamine, 97, 134
peperonal, 109
peppermint, 90, 98
perianal itching, 83, 117
peripheral vascular disease, 27, 54
permethrin, 108, 109, 114
phenothrin, 108, 109
phenylephrine, 133, 152
phenytoin, 97, 164
pholcodeine, 142
pimecrolimus, 175
piperazine, 117
pityriasis capitis see dandruff
podophyllum resin (podophyllin), 62-3
poloxamer '188', 70
polyvinyl acetate tear substitutes, 41
potassium bicarbonate antacids, 96, 98
potassium citrate, 194, 195
potassium-sparing diuretics, 194, 195
povidone-iodine, 166, 213
pregnancy, 58, 83, 158, 211, 212
   drug precautions/contraindications, 19, 25,
   27, 40, 63, 70, 85, 90, 99, 124, 151, 184, 195,
   204
premestrual syndrome, 207-10
prochlorperazine, 27
promethazine, 18, 142, 149, 176

propamidine isetionate, 39, 40
prostatic hypertrophy, 19, 27, 90, 142
pseudoephedrine, 133, 143
psoriasis, 48, 57, 175, 180
   scalp, 183, 184, 186, 187
pyridoxine, 207, 208-9
pyrithione zinc, 184, 185

raloxifene, 212
ranitidine, 98, 99
rectal prolapse, 84
reflux oesophagitis see gastro-oesophageal
   reflux (heartburn)
registration exam, 2-4
   question formats, 2-4
   structure, 2
renal disease, drug contraindications, 24, 27,
   71, 117, 195
resorcinol, 165, 166
Reye's syndrome, 25, 133, 199
rheumatoid arthritis, 38, 39, 42
rhinorrhoea (runny nose), 133-4, 148
RICE (rest, ice, compression and elevation),
   124
rifampicin, 97, 164
ringworm see tinea
rosacea, 164
rotavirus diarrhoea, 76
rubefacients (counterirritants), 125, 171

St John's wort, 27
salicylic acid, 48, 49, 50, 54-5, 62, 124, 125,
   165, 166, 184, 185, 187
scabies, 113-15
scalp conditions, 183-9
seborrhoeic dermatitis, 175, 183, 184, 185-6
seborrhoeic warts, 62
selenium sulphide, 181, 184
self-assessment
   acne, 167-8
   answers, 215-25
   athlete's foot, 50-1
   cardiovascular disease, 14
   cold sores, 171-2
   common cold, 136
   constipation, 73-4
   cough, 144-5
   cystitis, 195-6
   diarrhoea, 80-1
   dysmenorrhoea, 201
   ear problems, 35
   eczema/dermatitis, 177
   emergency hormonal contraception, 205
   eye conditions, 42-3
   foot (podiatric) problems, 56
   fungal skin infections, 181-2
   haemorrhoids, 86-7
   hayfever, 153

head lice, 110-11
indigestion, 100
influenza, 136-7
irritable bowel syndrome, 91
motion sickness, 20
mouth ulcers, 103
musculoskeletal conditions, 126-7
nicotine replacement therapy, 158-9
onychomycosis, 59
pain, 29
premenstrual syndrome, 209-10
scabies, 115
scalp conditions, 188-9
threadworm, 119
vaginal thrush, 214
warts/verrucas, 64
senna, 70, 117
sexually transmitted disease, 193
shingles, 21
silver nitrate, 63
simeticone, 98
simvastatin, 11-13
sinusitis, 21, 22, 148
skin
    fungal infection, 179-82
    tags, 62
smoking, 155
sodium bicarbonate, 34, 96, 98, 194
sodium cromoglycate, 151-2
sodium picosulfate, 70
sodium sulphate, 71
sore throat, 132, 134-5
spironolactone, 194, 195
sports injuries, 123
sprains, 123
squamous cell carcinoma, 62, 101
squill, 142
statins, 11-12
sterculia, 69
stimulant laxatives, 69-70
strains, 123
stroke, 10-11, 13
stye (hordeolum), 40-1
subarachnoid haemorrhage, 23
subconjunctival haemorrhage, 37
sulconazole, 48
sulfadiazine, 134
sulphur, 165, 166
sumatriptan, 26-7
sympathomimetic amines, 133, 143, 150, 152

tacrolimus, 175
tear substitutes (artificial tears), 41
temporal arteritis, 21, 23
tension headache, 21, 22, 26
terbinafine, 49, 58, 180
tetracyclines, 97, 167
theophylline, 95, 144, 158

threadworm, 117-19
throat lozenges/pastilles, 134-5, 144
thyroid disease, 68, 75, 133, 143
tinea
    capitis (scalp ringworm), 183, 187-8
    corporis (ringworm), 179-80
    cruris (dhobie/jock itch), 179, 180-1
    pedis see athlete's foot
tioconazole, 58
tolnaftate, 49
traction headache, 21
transient ischaemic attack, 10
traveller's diarrhoea, 75, 76, 80
trichomoniasis, 212
triclocarbon, 166
triclosan, 166
trigeminal neuralgia, 23, 28
trihexphenidyl (benzhexol), 68, 142
trimethoprim, 167, 195
triprolidine, 142
triptans, 26-7

ulcerative colitis, 38, 75, 89
undecenonic acid, 49
urea hydrogen peroxide, 34
urethral syndrome, 193
urinary frequency, 193
uveitis (iritis), 38

vaginal discharge, 194, 211, 212
vaginal thrush (vulvovaginal candidiasis),
    211-14
vascular headache, 21
verrucas, 61-4
viral conjunctivitis, 37, 39
viral cough, 139-40
vomiting/nausea, 17, 18, 27, 77-8, 200
vulvovaginal candidiasis (vaginal thrush),
    211-14

warfarin, 13, 25
warts, 61-4
Whitfield's ointment (Benzoic Acid Ointment
    Compound BP), 50
whooping cough (pertussis), 140

xylometazoline, 133, 152

zanamivir, 132
zinc oxide, 85
zinc sulphate, 171
zinc undecenoate, 49